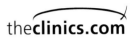

CRITICAL CARE NURSING CLINICS OF NORTH AMERICA

Monitoring and Hemodynamics

GUEST EDITOR
Barbara Leeper, MN, RN, CCRN

CONSULTING EDITOR
Suzanne S. Prevost, PhD, RN

June 2006 • Volume 18 • Number 2

SAUNDERS

An Imprint of Elsevier, Inc.
PHILADELPHIA   LONDON   TORONTO   MONTREAL   SYDNEY   TOKYO

W.B. SAUNDERS COMPANY
A Division of Elsevier Inc.

Elsevier Inc., 1600 John F. Kennedy Blvd., Suite 1800, Philadelphia, PA 19103-2899.

http://www.theclinics.com

CRITICAL CARE NURSING CLINICS OF NORTH AMERICA   **Volume 18, Number 2**
June 2006   **ISSN 0899-5885**
Editor: Ali Gavenda   **ISBN 1-4160-3503-6**

The ideas and opinions expressed in *Critical Care Nursing Clinics of North America* do not necessarily reflect those of the Publisher. The Publisher does not assume any responsibility for any injury and/or damage to persons or property arising out of or related to any use of the material contained in this periodical. The reader is advised to check the appropriate medical literature and the product information currently provided by the manufacturer of each drug to be administered to verify the dosage, the method and duration of administration, or contraindications. It is the responsibility of the treating physician or other health care professional, relying on independent experience and knowledge of the patient, to determine drug dosages and the best treatment for the patient. Mention of any product in this issue should not be construed as endorsement by the contributors, editors, or the Publisher of the product or manufacturers' claims.

Critical Care Nursing Clinics of North America (ISSN 0899-5885) is published quarterly by W.B. Saunders, 360 Park Avenue South, New York, NY 10010-1710. Months of publication are March, June, September, and December. Business and Editorial Offices: 1600 John F. Kennedy Blvd., Suite 1800, Philadelphia, PA 19103-2899. Accounting and Circulation Offices: 6277 Sea Harbor Drive, Orlando, FL 32887-4800. Periodicals postage paid at New York, NY and additional mailing offices. Subscription prices are $105.00 per year for US individuals, $175.00 per year for US institutions, $55.00 per year for US students and residents, $135.00 per year for Canadian individuals, $215.00 per year for Canadian institutions, $145.00 per year for international individuals, $215.00 per year for international institutions and $75.00 per year for Canadian and foreign students/residents. To receive student/resident rate, orders must be accompanied by name of affiliated institution, date of term, and the *signature* of program/residency coordinator on institution letterhead. Orders will be billed at individual rate until proof of status is received. Foreign air speed delivery is included in all *Clinics* subscription prices. All prices are subject to change without notice. **POSTMASTER:** Send address changes to *Critical Care Nursing Clinics of North America,* Elsevier Periodicals Customer Service, 6277 Sea Harbor Drive, Orlando, FL 32887-4800. **Customer Service: 1-800-654-2452 (US). From outside of the US, call 1-407-345-4000.**

Critical Care Nursing Clinics of North America is covered in *International Nursing Index, Nursing Citation Index, Cumulative Index to Nursing and Allied Health Literature,* and *RNdex Top 100.*

Printed in the United States of America.

GOAL STATEMENT

The goal of *Critical Care Nursing Clinics of North America* is to keep practicing critical care nurses up to date with current critical care clinical practice by providing timely articles reviewing the state of the art in critical care.

ACCREDITATION

Critical Care Nursing Clinics of North America is planned and implemented in accordance with the Essential Areas and Policies of the Accreditation Council for Continuing Medical Education (ACCME) through the joint sponsorship of the University of Virginia School of Medicine and Elsevier. The University of Virginia School of Medicine is accredited by the ACCME to provide continuing medical education for physicians.

The University of Virginia School of Medicine designates this educational activity for a maximum of 15 AMA PRA Category 1 Credits™. Physicians should only claim credit commensurate with the extent of their participation in the activity.
NOTE: The American Nurses Credentialing Center (ANCC), and many State Boards accept AMA category 1 credit issued by an ACCME provider to maintain ANA certifications or licensure. 15 AMA category 1 credits are equivalent to 18 ANA contact hours.

The American Medical Association has determined that physicians not licensed in the US who participate in this CME activity are eligible for 15 AMA PRA Category 1 Credits™.

Category 1 credit can be earned by reading the text material, taking the CME examination online at http://www.theclinics.com/home/cme, and completing the evaluation. After taking the test, you will be required to review any and all incorrect answers. Following completion of the test and evaluation, your credit will be awarded and you may print your certificate.

NOTE: The American Nurses Credentialing Center (ANCC), and many State Boards accept AMA category 1

FACULTY DISCLOSURE/CONFLICT OF INTEREST

The University of Virginia School of Medicine, as an ACCME accredited provider, endorses and strives to comply with the Accreditation Council for Continuing Medical Education (ACCME) Standards of Commercial Support, Commonwealth of Virginia statutes, University of Virginia policies and procedures, and associated federal and private regulations and guidelines on the need for disclosure and monitoring of proprietary and financial interests that may affect the scientific integrity and balance of content delivered in continuing medical education activities under our auspices.

The University of Virginia School of Medicine requires that all CME activities accredited through this institution be developed independently and be scientifically rigorous, balanced and objective in the presentation/discussion of its content, theories and practices.

All authors/editors participating in an accredited CME activity are expected to disclose to the readers relevant financial relationships with commercial entities occurring within the past 12 months (such as grants or research support, employee, consultant, stock holder, member of speakers bureau, etc.). The University of Virginia School of Medicine will employ appropriate mechanisms to resolve potential conflicts of interest to maintain the standards of fair and balanced education to the reader. Questions about specific strategies can be directed to the Office of Continuing Medical Education, University of Virginia School of Medicine, Charlottesville, Virginia.

The authors/editors listed below have identified no professional or financial affiliations for themselves or their spouse/partner:
Richard Arbour, RN, MSN, CCRN, CNRN; Elaine Button, RN, CDE; Sonya Flanders, RN, BSN, CCRN; Marjorie Funk, RN, PhD; Kathleen M. Hill, RN, MSN, CCNS; Patty Keaton, RN, BSN, CCRN; Deborah G. Klein, RN, BSN, MSN, CCRN, CS; JoAnne Phillips, MSN, RN, CCRN, CCNS; Donna Prentice, APRN, BC, CCRN; Marilyn Sommers, MD; Carrie Sona, APRN, BC, CCRN; Marita Titler, PhD, RN, FAAN; and Karen Zwerneman, MSN, RN, CCRN.

The authors listed below have not provided disclosure for themselves or their spouse/partner:
Nancy M. Albert, PhD, RN, CCNS, CCRN, CNA is an independent contractor for Cardiodynamics.
Mary Kay Bader, RN, MSN, CCRN, CNRN is on the speaker's bureau for Integra Neuroscience.
Barbara J. Drew, RN, PhD receives research support from Medtronic Emergency Response Systems, is on the speaker's bureau for GE and Philips, and is on the advisory committee for GE.
Cindy Goodrich, RN, MS, CCRN is a consultant and is on the speaker's bureau for Edwards Lifesciences.
Jan M. Headley, RN, BS is employed by and has stock in Edwards Lifesciences.
Barbara Leeper, MN, RN, CCRN is on the speaker's bureau for Edwards Lifesciences.

Disclosure of Discussion of non-FDA approved uses for pharmaceutical products and/or medical devices:
The University of Virginia School of Medicine, as an ACCME provider, requires that all faculty presenters identify and disclose any "off label" uses for pharmaceutical and medical device products. The University of Virginia School of Medicine recommends that each physician fully review all the available data on new products or procedures prior to instituting them with patients.

TO ENROLL

To enroll in the Critical Care Nursing Clinics of North America Continuing Medical Education program, call customer service at 1-800-654-2452 or visit us online at **www.theclinics.com/home/cme**. The CME program is available to subscribers for an additional fee of $99.00

CONSULTING EDITOR

SUZANNE S. PREVOST, PhD, RN, Nursing Professor and National HealthCare Chair of Excellence, Middle Tennessee State University, School for Nursing, Murfreesboro, Tennessee

EDITORIAL BOARD

GUEST EDITOR

BARBARA LEEPER, MN, RN, CCRN, Clinical Nurse Specialist, Cardiovascular Services, Baylor University Medical Center, Dallas, Texas

CONTRIBUTORS

NANCY M. ALBERT, PhD, CCNS, CCRN, CNA, Director, Nursing Research and Innovation, Division of Nursing; Clinical Nurse Specialist, Department of Cardiovascular Medicine, George M. and Linda H. Kaufman Center for Heart Failure, Cleveland Clinic, Cleveland, Ohio

RICHARD ARBOUR, RN, MSN, CCRN, CNRN, Staff Nurse/Clinical Researcher, Albert Einstein Healthcare Network, Philadelphia, Pennsylvania

MARY KAY BADER, RN, MSN, CCRN, CNRN, Neuro/Critical Care CNS, Mission Hospital, Mission Viejo, California

ELAINE BUTTON, RN, CDE, Director, Inpatient Diabetes Services, Healthways at Moses Cone Health System, Greensboro, South Carolina

BARBARA J. DREW, RN, PhD, Professor of Nursing and Clinical Professor of Medicine, School of Nursing, University of California, San Francisco, San Francisco, California

SONYA A. FLANDERS, RN, BSN, CCRN, Cardiovascular Nurse Clinician, Baylor University Medical Center, Dallas, Texas

MARJORIE FUNK, RN, PhD, Professor, School of Nursing, Yale University, New Haven, Connecticut

CINDY GOODRICH, RN, MS, CCRN, Flight Nurse, Airlift Northwest, Seattle, Washington

JAN M. HEADLEY, RN, BS, Director, Clinical Marketing and Professional Education, Edwards Lifesciences LLC, Irvine, California

KATHLEEN M. HILL, MSN, RN, CCNS, Clinical Nurse Specialist, Cardiothoracic Intensive Care Units, Cleveland Clinic, Cleveland, Ohio

PATTY KEATON, RN, BSN, CCRN, Moses Cone Health System, Greensboro, South Carolina

DEBORAH G. KLEIN, MSN, RN, CCRN, CS, Clinical Nurse Specialist, Cardiac Intensive Care Unit and Heart Failure Special Care Unit, Cleveland Clinic; Clinical Instructor, Frances Payne Bolton School of Nursing, Case Western Reserve University, Cleveland, Ohio

JOANNE PHILLIPS, MSN, RN, CCRN, CCNS, Clinical Nurse Specialist, Patient Safety, The Hospital of the University of Pennsylvania, Philadelphia, Pennsylvania

DONNA PRENTICE, APRN, BC, CCRN, Clinical Nurse Specialist, Medical Intensive Care Unit, Barnes-Jewish Hospital, St. Louis, Missouri

CARRIE SONA, APRN, BC, CCRN, Clinical Nurse Specialist, Surgical/Trauma Intensive Care Unit, Barnes-Jewish Hospital, St. Louis, Missouri

KAREN ZWERNEMAN, MSN, RN, CCRN, Director, Neurology, Vasular, & Renal Services, Baylor University Medical Center, Dallas, Texas

CONTENTS

CONTENTS

FORTHCOMING ISSUES

RECENT ISSUES

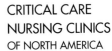
Preface

Monitoring and Hemodynamics

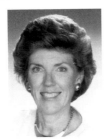

Barbara "Bobbi" Leeper, MN, RN, CCRN
Guest Editor

Monitoring is an integral component of patient care, regardless of location. The articles in this issue offer different approaches to improving patient outcomes using various monitoring technologies.

The availability of additional devices for monitoring has led to the addition of more alarms in the clinical setting. The challenge for practitioners is responding to alarms. Often the alarms may not be heard, or in the worst-case scenario, may be ignored due to sensory overload, potentially resulting in negative patient outcomes. As a result the Joint Commission on Hospital Accreditation Organization (JCAHO) became interested in this issue. Phillips, in her article, *Clinical Alarms: Complexity and Common Sense*, discusses alarm safety, how to perform an environmental assessment for clinical alarms, issues surrounding alarm responses, and recommendations for an alarm safety program.

Continuous EKG monitoring has been in existence for more than 40 years, however, it is only recently that standards for this practice have been published. Drew and Funk provide an executive summary on key elements of the standards and address some challenges that may occur with implementation. One large component of those standards is the use of continuous ST-segment monitoring. Flanders discusses the clinical applicability of continuous ST-segment monitoring, addressing specific patient populations in which

this technology has proven to be helpful in improving patient outcomes.

Monitoring the balance between oxygen delivery and tissue oxygen demand is an integral component of monitoring the critically ill. The technology may assess this balance on a global basis or on a more regional basis. Cardiac output monitoring is one aspect of oxygen delivery. There is a trend in cardiac output monitoring toward moving away from invasive technologies to the use of less-invasive or non-invasive technology. Three articles in this issue address different types of less-invasive or non-invasive cardiac output monitoring technologies, including the use of arterial pulse wave cardiac output, esophageal Doppler monitoring, and finally, bioimpedence cardiography. All three articles offer insights into the incorporation of these technologies into clinical practice in the ICU, as well as outside the ICU environment.

Goodrich provides a comprehensive review of the literature on the use of a newer global parameter, continuous venous oximetry monitoring in the superior vena cava, which can be used as a surrogate for mixed venous oxygen saturation. Hill and Klein introduce the technology of continuous transcutaneous pCO_2 monitoring, which early studies indicate to be beneficial in the early identification of respiratory failure when compared to continuous pulse oximetry. Zwerneman discusses the importance and use of end-

doi:10.1016/j.ccell.2006.03.001

tidal CO_2 monitoring. Bader describes the potential application of brain tissue oxygen ($PbtO_2$) monitoring technology in the care of traumatic brain-injured and subarrachnoid hemorrhage patients.

The final two articles address important issues on monitoring from a different perspective. Arbour evaluates the correlation between the bispectral index (BIS) and clinical assessment of sedation, and discusses differences in outcomes between patients monitored using the BIS concurrent with clinical assessment and patients monitored using clinical assessment alone. Button and Keaton demonstrate the effectiveness of glycemic control in coronary artery bypass graft patients with the use of IV insulin regulated by a computerized system. The use of these technologies provides us with more information than ever before, offering clinicians a better picture of patient physiology and a real opportunity to improve outcomes.

Barbara "Bobbi" Leeper, MN, RN, CCRN
Cardiovascular Services
Baylor University Medical Center
3500 Gaston Avenue
Dallas, TX 75246, USA
E-mail address: bobbil@baylorhealth.edu

ELSEVIER
SAUNDERS

Crit Care Nurs Clin N Am 18 (2006) 145 – 156

CRITICAL CARE
NURSING CLINICS
OF NORTH AMERICA

Clinical Alarms: Complexity and Common Sense

JoAnne Phillips, MSN, RN, CCRN, CCNS

The Hospital of the University of Pennsylvania, 3400 Spruce Street, Philadelphia, PA, 19104, USA

In 2002, the Joint Commission on Accreditation of Health Care Organizations (JCAHO) reviewed 23 reports of death or injury that were related to mechanical ventilation. Nineteen of those events resulted in death, and 4 resulted in coma; 65% were related to alarms. The issues included delayed or no response to the alarm; the alarm was off or set incorrectly; no alarms for certain types of ventilator disconnections; or the alarm was not audible in all areas of patient care [1]. This review prompted JCAHO to include alarm safety in the National Patient Safety Goals (NPSG) for 2003. For clinicians, assessing clinical alarm systems was a complex undertaking. Where should one start? How in-depth should one look? What are the implications for the findings? Was it all just common sense? This article examines the components of an alarm safety program, from the complex to the common sense.

Alarm safety

Effective January 1, 2003 all health care organizations were required to comply with a two-part NPSG on clinical alarms. The first part of the goal was to improve the effectiveness of clinical alarm systems by implementing regular preventive maintenance and testing of alarm systems. The second part of the goal was to assure that alarms were activated with appropriate settings to notify clinicians of a change in clinical condition or a dysfunction of a piece of equipment. The goal also stated that alarms were audible with respect to distances and competing noise within the unit (ie, could the alarm be heard on the

unit where it is sounding during the normal daily activities of the unit?) [2].

Although the risk was assessed through the review of ventilator-associated events, the goal was global and referred to all clinical alarm systems in the patient care arena. Attention to clinical alarm systems, particularly the requirement for assuring activation, proper settings, and audibility, had not received a high level of interest until it was part of a NPSG [3]. Beginning in 2005, however, JCAHO no longer considered Clinical Alarms a NPSG, it is now a standard in the Environment of Care Standards. Over those 2 years, the complexity of alarms systems was examined with renewed appreciation. This article guides the acute care team through the evaluation of the clinical environment as it relates to alarm systems. Key components in an alarm system evaluation and risk assessment are presented to guide the clinicians in assessing current systems or future alarm system purchases. There also is a discussion of an alarm safety program, including key aspects of policy development and educational and competency validation resources.

Clinical alarms: environmental assessment

A clinical alarm is a notification from a device that is used to diagnose, treat, or monitor a patient. It is an audible or visual alert to the clinician that the patient's physiologic parameter has exceeded the set limits or that there is an equipment malfunction. All alarms are designed to alert clinicians that a change has occurred that requires attention. In assessing the clinical area for alarms, nursing must establish a partnership with the clinical engineering team. Their expertise in understanding the mechanical operation

E-mail address: joanne.phillips@uphs.upenn.edu

146

PHILLIPS

of each piece of equipment is invaluable to assessing the patient care environment. Environmental assessments must be completed on each unit that is being assessed to appreciate fully the ambient environmental distractions. Within that environment, there are many alarms that are not directly patient centered. These are alarms that need to be answered, but they may not affect the clinical aspect of patient care immediately. Examples of those alarms include the fire alarm or the pneumatic tube system (used for delivery of supplies and medications). Assessment also includes patient-centered alarms (eg, infusion pumps, feeding pumps, mechanical ventilators, physiologic monitors, nurse call lights). The number of patient-centered alarms can be overwhelming.

In assessing the multitude of patient-centered alarms in a clinical area, not all alarms are equally important. In 2001, Chambrin and colleagues [4] published classifications from the European Committee on Standardization that delineated alarms as high, medium, and low priority. High-priority alarms indi-

cate an urgent situation that requires immediate attention; medium-priority alarms indicate a dangerous situation that requires a quick response, and low priority alarms indicate that attention is needed. In a similar model, which was developed at the Hospital of the University of Pennsylvania, an environmental assessment led to the development of a system in which all alarms in a clinical area were classified as level I, II, or III (Fig. 1). The importance of delineating alarm response relates to the risk that is associated with that individual alarm. If that alarm goes unanswered, what are the potential clinical implications? Clinical environments may have 40 alarm sources, possibly more in certain areas [4].

Most alarms in the clinical areas are auditory. Nurses may perceive themselves as experts at discerning which alarms are sounding, but several studies dispute that belief. Cropp and colleagues [5] audiotaped 33 sounds in an ICU. The nurses identified the sources of the sounds correctly only 50% of the time. When alarms sound the same, it is difficult

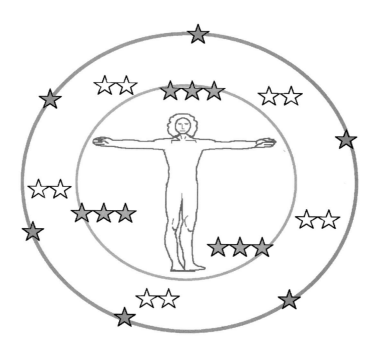

Fig. 1. Constellation man.
    Level I: (1 star): requires intervention
    Examples: feeding pump; air mattress
    Level II: (2 stars): requires rapid intervention
    Examples: level II cardiac alarm; nurse call lights
    Level III: (3 stars): requires immediate retention
    Examples: ventilator disconnect; ventricular fibrillation
    INOP: Monitoring is inoperative (cardiac leads are off)
(Courtesy of The Hospital of the University of Pennsylvania; with permission.)

to differentiate the source of the alarm and the criticality of that alarm [6]. Auditory alarms, which are relied on to notify us of significant clinical events, have been designed inadequately; there is a poor match between the importance of an alarm and how it sounds [7].

In the operating room, auditory alarms substantially increase the speed and appropriateness of the response by the anesthesia care provider. The goal in alarm design is to create an alarm that is instantly recognizable by the trained respondent. Recommendations from the International Organization on Standardization state that an alarm with a high pitch and rapid repetition is perceived as more urgent than is a sound with a lower pitch or slower repetition [8]. Although humans comply better with auditory alarms than visual alarms [9], they have difficulty with reliably differentiating more than six alarms at a time [10]. Newer monitoring systems, with "intelligent alarms," are much more efficient at helping the staff to differentiate alarms.

Alarm response

Appropriate alarm response is a complex, yet vital, standard for all patient care units. Often, the bedside care providers are the least experienced clinicians and are responsible for assessing and responding to alarms [11]. Several factors (eg, high nurse workload, ergonomics of the room/unit design, unit culture) influence alarm response. Culture is a shared set of beliefs and values about how people work individually and in teams. Culture dictates rules, norms, and behaviors. It also influences how one behaves in a particular situation. Unit policies—coupled with unit culture—define alarm response. Criteria for alarm setting and customization for individual patients, defeating alarms, and silencing alarms must be defined clearly [12]. Responsibility and accountability for alarm response also must be delineated clearly. The leadership on each unit must create a culture that integrates the nonpatient-centered alarms and the patient-centered alarms into a culture of patient safety that is reflected in daily practice. Every nurse is responsible for every alarm. This cultural norm is especially important outside of the ICU, where nurse/patient ratios tend to be higher and the geography of the units may not support easy visibility of patients. Stand-alone monitors, which are more likely to be present on general care floors, present a particular risk. A clear policy about where to locate patients with respect to the audibility of critical alarms is essential [13]. For example, a patient

with a stand-alone pulse oximeter must be located near the nurses' station—with the door open at all times—to assure audibility of the alarm. The locations of patients who are receiving medications on infusion pumps also must be evaluated critically.

The complexity of our clinical environment requires the establishment of a tiered alarm response; this ensure that if the primary caregiver is attending to another patient a back-up person can attend to the alarm [14]. For example, if a two-star alarm sounds in a telemetry pager system and it is not responded to in a prescribed period of time, that alarm should be sent automatically to another nurse, often the charge nurse. Alarms may sound as often as every 30 seconds in a critical care unit [15]. Thus, the criticality of the alarms must be delineated to establish the level of response. Using a system of alarm levels (see Fig. 1) helps the staff to understand the criticality of each alarm.

To respond appropriately, the nurse must understand the implications for each alarm. There are various reasons why alarms are not responded to appropriately. In addition to the factors that were mentioned earlier, the nurse may be caring for other patients, the alarm for one patient may not be audible in another patient's room, the alarm may not be set appropriately, or the importance of that alarm may not be recognized. Staffing and training issues also may play a role [10]. The overwhelming numbers of nuisance or low-level alarms also play key roles in alarm response. There are several consequences of too many false or low-priority alarms. If an alarm is perceived to be reliable 90% of the time, it is responded to more than 90% of the time. If it is perceived to be reliable 10% of the time, it will be responded to 10% of the time. It is unlikely that the 10% of alarms that are responded to are those that are meaningful. Alarm systems are almost useless when false alarm rates are high [9]. Overwhelming the ambient environment with alarms makes normal communication difficult. These clinically irrelevant alarms distract staff from what they are doing, which increases the chance for an error. Most importantly, the more nuisance alarms that sound, the more likely it is that the staff will ignore the alarms—and potentially—a clinically relevant alarm [9].

To address the alarm response issue, some institutions have introduced the concept of "alarm drills." The Environment of Care Committee at Valley Regional Hospital in Claremont, New Hampshire introduced the concept of alarm drills. The hospital policy requires the establishment of a list of all of the equipment in the hospital that has a critical clinical alarm. A baseline response of how quickly staff

Table 1
WakeMed Assessment Tool used for The Hospital of the University of Pennsylvania clinical alarm assessment

Alarm type	Person responsible PM	Audibility test	Response Policy covering response	Setting limits Policy covering setting alarms	Central alarm	Central silence	Problem area/action plan/priority status
Emergency light	CE		Nursing staff	NA	Yes	No	
Nurse call light	CE		Nursing staff	NA	Yes	Yes	
Mechanical ventilator	CE		RN/RT: mechanical ventilator	RT: Mechanical Ventilator	No	No	
Cardiac alarms Level III	CE		RN Procedure for Cardiac Monitoring: 4B-04-1	RN Procedure for Cardiac Monitoring: 4B-04-1	Yes	Yes	
Cardiac alarms Level II	CE						
Cardiac alarms Level I/leads off	CE						
Arterial pressure monitor	CE		RN: Hemodynamic Monitoring	RN: Hemodynamic Monitoring	No	No	
Pneumatic tube	Physical plant		All staff	NA	Yes	Yes	
Prisma machine	Gambro Renal Services		RN staff: CRRT	Preset	No	No	
IV pumps	CE		RN Alaris Pump Policy: 4B-02-09	Preset by CE RN sets rate, volume, dose	No	No	
Transport monitor	CE		RN: Cardiac Monitoring: 4B-04-1	RN: Cardiac Monitoring: 4B-04-1	No	No	
Medical gas	CE		RN/RT: Utility and Medical Gas Failure Guidelines for Patient Care Units: 4B-01-16	Physical plant	Yes	No	

Abbreviations: Alarm limit setting, who sets the alarms; Alarm response, primary responsibility to respond to alarm; Audibility testing, ensuring alarm is audible on specific unit; CE, clinical engineering; Central alarm, does alarm sound at central station; Central Silence, is it possible to silence alarm at central station; CRRT, Continuous renal replacement therapy; NA, Not Applicable; Nursing staff, Registered nurse and certified nursing assistant; PM, Preventive maintenance; RT, Respiratory therapy. (Courtesy of WakeMed, Wake County, North Carolina; with permission.)

should respond to each clinical alarm was established. After the baseline was established, the environment of care team conducted alarm drills to assess appropriate response to alarms. A positive response during the drill means that the nurse arrives at the bedside, knows why the alarm is sounding, and responds appropriately to rectify the alarm. A failed response is one in which the nurse fails to arrive within the predetermined time frame or does not know why the alarm is sounding or what steps to take to rectify the alarm. A failed response results in the staff receiving education on alarm safety and a repeated drill in 3 months [15]. Alarm drills are one strategy to evaluate staff response; there may be other effective strategies.

True or false?

The activation of clinical alarms is essential in notifying clinicians of a change in the clinical status of a patient or the malfunction of a piece of equipment. Many clinical environments are subject to a multitude of alarms that are of no clinical significance. Alarms can be classified as true and clinically relevant, true and clinically irrelevant, or false. True and clinically relevant indicates that an alarm sounds in response to a clinical change that prompts an intervention (eg, a patient develops supraventricular tachycardia and his heart rate goes up to 200 beats/min, which is 40 beats greater than the high limit). A transient increase in blood pressure during a suctioning event is an example of a true and clinically irrelevant event. An alarm sounds, but it is clinically irrelevant and the parameter will go back to baseline without treatment. A false alarm is an alarm that sounds because the alarm parameters were violated, but that violation was not part of the clinical presentation (Keller J. Implementing safety-based clinical alarm strategies. ECRI perspectives 2003; March: Audioconference). Often, false alarms are referred to as nuisance alarms. An example is a cardiac monitor that alarms for "irregular rhythm" for patients who have chronic atrial fibrillation. The rhythm is irregular, but it is the baseline rhythm for that patient. Another example is the frequent loss of signal from a pulse oximeter probe if the probe falls off. Frequent false alarms cause the staff to ignore, disable, or silence alarm devices [4]. In evaluating the plethora of alarms that occur in critical care units, several studies showed that less than 10% of alarms induce a therapeutic modification [4;Keller J. Implementing safety-based clinical alarm strategies. ECRI perspectives 2003; March: Audioconference]. In one study,

alarms that were associated with patient intervention (eg, suctioning, repositioning) occurred four times more often than did alarms that were not associated with patient intervention. False positive alarms (an alarm that sounds for a value that does not reflect the patient's condition) occur as often with intervention (82%) as with nonintervention (86%) [16]. These

Table 2
Alarm risk assessment

Activity	Key components
Develop matrix of all medical alarms	Identify the purpose for the alarm
	Identify hardware/software components
	Human factors related to setting, responding to, and managing the alarm while in use
	Determine where the equipment will be used, who will use it, who will be responsible for preventive maintenance
	Use "WakeMed" tool to summarize data
Determine the potential severity of alarm-related issues on patient outcomes	Search FDA MAUDE database for outcomes from alarm-related issues
	Perform a failure mode and effects analysis to determine risk of clinical alarm systems
Identification of environmental factors that would effect audibility	Evaluate whether the design of the alarm needs to be changed
	Evaluate whether patients with particular devices need to be located strategically to facilitate audibility
	Evaluate whether particular devices should be restricted to particular units/geographic areas within a particular unit
Assessment of field experience to determine if there is a history of device-related problems in the literature or reported to the Food and Drug Administration (FDA) or other reporting organization	Search FDA MAUDE database and other databases for issues with particular devices

Adapted from Keil O. Managing medical alarms: a pratical approach to meeting the JCAHO National Safety Patient Goal. Available at: http://www.clinicaldynamics.com/downloads/test_report_revB.pdf.

studies noted that no major clinical compromise occurred without alarm notification. This suggests that current clinical monitoring is effective in notifying clinicians of a physiologic change or equipment malfunction, but is fraught with an overwhelming number of nuisance alarms. Over time, staff can become desensitized to alarms. This may lead to the staff ignoring, disabling, or silencing the alarms [4]. Another risk is that the staff may set the limits so broadly that they are unlikely to be exceeded [14].

Although most alarm studies have been conducted in critical care settings, alarms in intermediate care and general care areas are of particular concern. These areas tend to have lower nurse/patient ratios with architectural layouts that are not conducive to audibility of the important alarms. Renewed attention to the risk that is associated with clinical alarms has occurred since the inception of the NPSG on clinical alarms.

Alarm system assessments

Alarm systems are an integral part of every clinical environment. To standardize the assessment—whether evaluating a critical care unit, an emergency department, or a general care floor—begin by establishing an inventory of devices/systems within the clinical environment that have alarms. Examples include physiologic monitors, infusion pumps, balloon pumps, elopement alarms, and mechanical ventilators. This is accomplished best with a partnership between clinical engineering and nursing. Table 1 is a practical tool that was developed by WakeMed. It concisely defines each alarm in the inventory, and delineates who is responsible for the testing, which policies define alarm response and limit setting, whether the alarm sounds centrally, or whether the alarm is able to be silenced centrally. It also facilitates feedback on alarm issues to the staff on

---

Box 1. Clinical alarm assessment

Clinical alarm assessment

Unit_____Date of Evaluation_____Patient Population_____ Inpt / Outpt

Critical Alarms:

☐ Hard wire monitors ☐ Telemetry monitors ☐ Telemetry beepers

☐ IV Pumps ☐ CVVH ☐ Feeding pumps ☐ IABP ☐ Call light beepers

☐LVAD / BiVAD ☐_____ ☐_____ ☐_____

☐_____ ☐_____ ☐_____ ☐_____

Cardiac alarms

Default alarms:

Heart Rate: High ☐_____ Low ☐_____

Arterial BP: High ☐_____ Low ☐_____

Noninvasive BP: High ☐_____ Low ☐_____

Pulse oximetry: Low ☐_____

Are any arrhythmias turned off (eg, R on T) _____

Do you know if all the default alarms in the monitors are the same?_____

Who decides on the alarm limits/arrhythmia? _____

How are the limits communicated?_____

How are the alarms documented?_____

Are the audible alarms on in the rooms?_____

What is the current practice on overview alarms? _____

What is the current practice for alarm review? _____

What is the standard for documentation?_____

The Hospital of the University of Pennsylvania

BP, blood pressure, IV, intravenous.

Abbreviations: Inpt, inpatient; Outpt, Outpatient; IABP, Intra-aortic balloon pump; LVAD/BIVAD, Left ventricular assist device/biventricular assist device; R on T is an alarm setting.
Courtesy of The Hospital of the University of Pennsylvania; with permission.

Box 2. Alarm activation and practice assessment [21]

Does the equipment alarm centrally and at the bedside?

Is there any equipment that has alarm enhancements? One example is the mechanical ventilator, which may be connected to the central monitor through several different types of devices (eg, a Vue-link Module from Philips Medical, Andover, MA).

Silencing and disabling: what are the current practices and are they safe? Does the staff understand the difference between silence and suspend on the monitor?

Are alarms silenced inappropriately from the central station? Is there a policy that addresses which alarms can and cannot be silenced at the central station (eg, high priority or leads off alarms)?

What is the unit culture on alarm response?

Does the staff understand the alarm chain priority in the cardiac alarm system?

Are the alarms latched (continues to alarm until it is responded to) or unlatched (stops alarming when the violation has stopped)?

By activating all alarms within a clinical environment, are there any alarms that are not audible/visible at the central nurse's station?

How are alarms communicated: audible in the unit; remote telemetry monitors; cell phones; pagers?

Does the unit have patient care areas (eg, a physical therapy gym or a classroom where patients attend class) that are physically associated with the unit where patients may be attending sessions? Does each of these areas have a ''panic button'' to notify the nursing unit of an emergency?

What is the expectation of alarm response (unit culture)? Is the responsibility for alarm response delineated clearly?

How are the alarm settings communicated from caregiver to caregiver?

Is alarm event review part of nurse to nurse shift report?

How does the nurse use the alarm event review to customize alarm settings?

What is the standard for documentation? Is that a consistent standard throughout the institution?

each unit. After the inventory is established, an alarm assessment should be conducted in each clinical area [12].

Integral to the completion of an alarm system assessment is evaluating the risk that is associated with clinical alarms. Table 2 delineates key components in a risk assessment tool [17]. Further assessment can be completed with the Clinical Alarm Assessment Tool (Boxes 1,2). This tool helps to define variation in practice from unit to unit. Unit-to-unit assessments may reveal inconsistent default settings or an inconsistent knowledge base on setting, defeating, and the customization of alarms. One of the goals of any safety program, including alarm safety, is to standardize practice across clinical environments. It is essential to conduct alarm assessments on each unit with the staff nurses and leadership of that unit. The staff nurse is at the sharp edge of patient safety, and is the person who is consistently closest to the patient. The staff nurse will be best able to describe the culture of alarm safety within each area.

After the inventory of devices/alarm systems has been established and the risk assessment is complete, the final component is the development of a practical testing plan. In collaboration with each unit leadership, the best time for device alarm testing and alarm system testing should be determined. All alarms must be tested at the busiest time of day, with devices as far from the nurses' station as is possible. This test ensures that the device or system is evaluated in a real clinical scenario, not in a testing laboratory. Testing includes activation of the alarm and assessment of the staff response to the alarm. Each piece of equipment requires a different approach. For example, areas to address when assessing a mechanical ventilator alarm include (1) verifying that the minute volume and low peak inspiratory alarms are set appropriately; (2) asking the staff to explain the hows and whys of ventilator alarm settings; (3) verifying adequate alarm volume, inside and outside of the room; (4) asking how was the nurse trained on the ventilator; (5) asking if there is a hospital policy on who can set the ventilator alarms; and (6) asking if there is a standard default for ventilator settings (Keller J. Implementing safety-based clinical alarm strategies. ECRI perspectives 2003; March: Audioconference). These questions can be the foundation of competent care for a patient who is on a mechanical ventilator, which should include an assessment of the nurse's knowledge of the alarm system on the ventilator. These concepts can be applied to other equipment with critical alarms, such as physiologic monitors, bedside dialysis machines, or infusion pumps.

Alarm system problems

To evaluate the effectiveness of a clinical alarm system, several components should be evaluated. Fig. 2 illustrates the complexity of alarm system

problems [18]. System problems include user error, physical layout/environment, technical issues, and miscellaneous issues. Analyzing the effect that each of these system problems has on the alarm system will guide the clinicians in developing an alarm safety program for each clinical environment.

Components of an alarm safety program

Establishing an alarm safety program is a complex process that involves many disciplines. In addition to the collaboration between clinical engineering and nursing, other disciplines (eg, respiratory therapy, facilities management) play a key role. An alarm safety program integrates a technology assessment and a clinical evaluation. One strategy to initialize an alarm safety program is to perform a failure mode and effects analysis, as defined by JCAHO [19]. This strat-

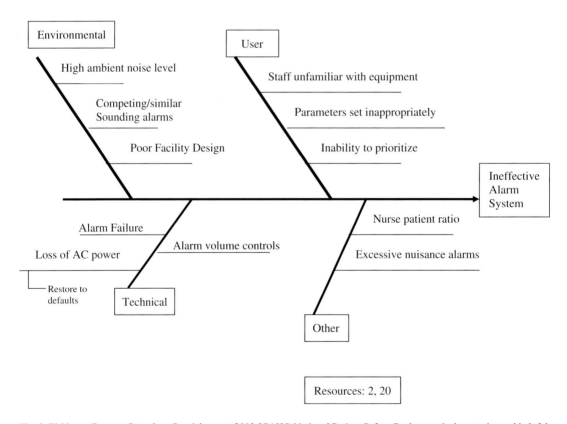

Fig. 2. Fishbone diagram. *Data from* Special report: 2003 JCAHO National Patient Safety Goals: practical strategies and helpful solutions for meeting these goals. Joint Commission Resources. Available at: http://www.jcrinc.com/subscribers/printview. asp?durki=3746; and Richardson W. Home study program: clinical alarm systems testing—a program assessment model. AORN J 2004;80(2):280–93.

egy will help each organization to define particular risks that are related to alarm safety.

Technology

Appropriate equipment selection is essential to the success of any alarm safety program. Different clinical areas have different needs, and equipment selection should match the clinical needs of the patients. Extra technology or monitoring is not beneficial to patients or staff when it provides information that is not helpful in clinical decision making, or may provide a distraction from the clinically relevant information. Table 3 provides a chart of 10 different alarm system components [20]. Although the focus of the components of this chart is for physiologic monitoring, the concepts can be applied when evaluating monitoring or therapeutic equipment for potential purchase.

After the technology is selected, or in evaluating current technology, several questions must be answered about default settings.

Are the alarm defaults the same on all like technology (eg, cardiac monitors; infusion pumps)?

Who decides what the default alarm limits should be?

Do all cardiac monitors have the same defaults? Are they appropriate for all clinical environments?

Does the staff know what the defaults are? Do steps need to be taken between patients to assure that the defaults are activated (eg, assuring the previous patient is discharged from the bedside and central stations)?

Is the overview feature (the ability to monitor a patient from a different patient's room) available and is it part of the defaults? Is it customizable to the individual unit's needs?

In establishing default settings, it is essential that all practitioners understand each alarm and the implications for violation. For example, some cardiac monitors have multiple premature ventricular contraction (PVC) alerts. The nurse needs to understand the criteria for each and what type of violation would initiate a high- or medium-level alarm. This knowledge would assist the clinicians in deciding on default settings. Many of the newer monitors count PVCs even if an alarm is not initiated; this may meet the clinical need to track the PVCs without creating a clinically irrelevant alarm.

After these questions are answered, and the matrix of equipment has been established, an alarm safety program can be developed. The important components of an alarm safety program include development of appropriate clinical policies, a process for validation of competency on alarm safety, and education and impact on practice at the bedside.

Clinical policies and competency validation

Integrating the components of alarm safety into a policy may seem to be straightforward; however, the challenge in changing policies is that every policy that discusses a piece of equipment with an alarm must be reviewed and revised to ensure that alarm response is addressed in each policy. Although most policies are under nursing, many are interdisciplinary. For example, the setting, defeating, silencing, or response to a ventilator alarm most often is a dual responsibility between nursing and respiratory therapy.

In developing an evidence-based approach to clinical alarms, a search of the literature did not produce a significant body of evidence on the setting, defeating, and silencing of alarms. Another important question is how to customize alarms to individual patients; this is not delineated well in the literature. This is essential in decreasing nuisance alarms, the risk of which was discussed earlier. An assessment of current practice may reveal a lack of knowledge of alarm defaults, alarm prioritization, and alarm response. This is of particular concern as it relates to cardiac monitors, because the alarm systems are extremely complex. Key components of a clinical policy that addresses alarms include:

Defining the criticality of alarms

Defining the setting and alarm response expectations, specifically addressing the leads-off or "INOP" alarm

Identifying other clinical policies that address alarms

Environmental considerations (eg, ambient noise, the use of stand-alone devices with critical alarms, alarm volume standards)

Lines of responsibility and accountability for alarm response

Testing of alarms

Nuisance alarms: strategies to decrease occurrence of nuisance alarms

Policy on cardiac monitoring that should include information about the criticality of each level of alarm

Table 3
Alarm system evaluation

Components	Description
Initialization of alarms	When the device is powered on, do the alarms sound immediately or when the patient is attached? By waiting until the patient is attached, it avoids nuisance alarms.
Prioritization	If the alarm is not answered in a prescribed period of time, does the alarm volume increase? Is the alarm sent to another beeper?
Alarm limits	How well can the limits be seen on the central display? Bedside display? If they cannot be seen, inappropriate alarm settings are less likely to be noticed by a clinician. When the monitor is turned off, do the alarm limits revert to the default limits? In certain systems, if the previous patient is not discharged from the monitor system, the original patient's settings will be maintained. Are the limits set by default, or does the monitor automatically set the limits based on the patient's physiologic parameters?
Volume	At the lowest setting, are the alarms audible? Can the alarm audibility be turned off at the bedside? For stand-alone monitors, can the alarm be heard outside the room? Even with the door closed?
Disabling and silencing	Is there a visual indicator that the alarm is silenced? What is the silence period? Is there a reminder that the alarm is silenced? What effect does that have on other alarms? If the clinician silences one alarm, will it affect other alarms? Does silencing one patients' alarm at the central station affect other patients' alarms? Can the audible "leads off" alarm be disabled for any reason? If the alarm has been silenced, does it stay silenced for an indeterminate period, until the alarm condition is rectified?
Systems alarms	Does the bedside unit alarm for weak battery (in those models that can undock from the bedside for transport)?
Arrhythmia alarms	Does the monitor have the ability to change the priority of lethal alarms? Can the central station prioritize lethal arrhythmias over nonlethal arrhythmias? Is arrhythmia processing done at the central station or in the bedside monitor?
Bed-to-bed notification	Are all alarms activated in other patients' rooms? Can the alarm be responded to remotely from another patient's room? Are they visual, audio or both? If the clinician silences the alarm from a remote location, will it silence it only at that remote location, or also at the central station and in the room where the violation occurred? Can the system be configured so that only low-level alarms can be silenced remotely? Can the system be configured so that only the highest level alarms can be heard in other patients' rooms? Can overview from room to room easily be activated temporarily? Can alarm groups be set up or changed easily? This is especially important when relying on beepers for alarm notification. Is there a limit to the number of beds that can integrate into one monitor? This may require the construction of alarm groupings in larger units.
Bedside device integration	Key question: what is the functionality of any bedside device integration when there is loss of signal from the bedside? What are the visual and audio presentations at the central station? Can ventilator alarms be integrated into the bedside monitor alarm system? If bedside devices are integrated and their alarm is silenced, is there a visual indicator that the integrated device is silenced? How are the integrated devices prioritized at the central station? If the bedside device is a ventilator, are the ventilator alarms prioritized appropriately? Are the ventilator alarms the same for the bedside and the central station? Do the ventilator alarms need to be set by the clinician after the device is integrated?
Leads off	Does the monitor use automatic ECG switching for leads off?

Data from Physiologic monitoring systems. Health Devices 2005;34(1):5–45.

> **Box 3. Development of competency on clinical alarms**
>
> Identifies clinically significant alarms within the practice environment
> Explains need for alarms to patient and family
> Stratifies responsibility for:
>   Setting clinical alarms
>   Responding to clinical alarms
> Collaborates with other staff to establish a tiered response to alarms
> Optimizes patient placement for audibility, especially of stand-alone alarms
> Participates with clinical engineering in the testing of alarms
> Responds appropriately to any clinical alarm within the practice environment

Event review (reviewing the previous shift's alarms with the oncoming shift) is essential to change the cultural norm to "customize alarms," rather than listening to an overwhelming number of clinically irrelevant alarms. In deciding how to customize the alarm settings, collaboration between the physician, nurse practitioner, and primary nurse is essential. Why is the patient on the cardiac monitor, pulse oximeter, or other monitor? Is it related to a medication that the patient is receiving? Does the patient have chronic premature ventricular contractions (PVCs) that are not treated? If so, the PVC alarm may be adjusted to sound only when there is a high number of consecutive PVCs (the number is customizable to each patient). To customize cardiac alarms, the nurse must be well-versed in the meaning of each alarm (eg, difference between ventricular tachycardia and a run of PVCs; what type of alarm would each initiate?). This is just one example of a critical alarm; our clinical areas contain a multitude of alarms, from a variety of sources.

The clinical policy can be used as the foundation for developing the competency, which is the integration of clinical knowledge and psychomotor performance.

Box 3 contains guidance on developing a clinical competency on clinical alarms.

After a clinical alarm policy has been developed, other clinical policies that address equipment with alarms have been reviewed and revised, and the competency has been developed, an educational program must be constructed. Box 4 describes an educational program that addresses that need. The program should be focused on all bedside care providers, including nurses, nursing assistants, respiratory therapists, and any other direct care provider who may have responsibility for alarm response. The self-learning module is an essential component to providing a foundation of consistent information for the staff.

Metrics of success

The level of success may be difficult to measure. A review of the nursing flow sheets demonstrates the compliance with the documentation of alarm settings, and possibly a collaborative discussion on the appropriate alarm setting for individual patients.

> **Box 4. Educational program**
>
> Overview of alarm project
> Assessment strategies
>   Wake Medical Center assessment
>   Equipment inventory
>   Recommendations to physical plant/clinical engineering/administration
> Educational components
>   Lead placement
>   Lead selection
>   Unit-specific default
>   Alarm parameter review
>   Customization of alarms
>   Root cause of "leads off"
>   Competency on clinical alarms
> Resources
>   Self-learning module
>   Competencies:
>   Cardiac monitoring
>   Clinical alarms
>   Policies
>   Clinical alarms
>   Cardiac monitoring and alarm response
>   Alarm configuration tool

Summary

Clinical alarms serve an essential role in the clinical environment; they notify clinicians of a change in physiology or a malfunction of a piece of equipment. The ever-increasing number of these alarms is overwhelming the ambient environment with clinically irrelevant noise. It is essential to make alarms as meaningful as possible by eliminating nuisance alarms and by assuring that patients have an appropriate level of monitoring [5]. This will be particularly important in the future because our environments will have more alarms, no matter how many nuisance alarms are eliminated. Alarm enhancements for stand-alone equipment (eg, ventilators) will become more common. To increase the efficiency of alarms systems we must standardize warning sounds from system to system, and design alarms systems in which the urgency of alarm sounds is related to the criticality of the alarm. We must assess the complex, and translate it to common sense.

References

[1] Sentinel events alert: preventing ventilator related deaths and injuries. Available at: http://www.jcaho.org/about+us/news+letters/sentinel+event+alert/print/sea_25.htm. Accessed September 22, 2005.

[2] Special report: 2003 JCAHO National Patient Safety Goals: practical strategies and helpful solutions for meeting these goals. Joint Commission Resources. Available at: http://www.jcrinc.com/subscribers/printview.asp?durki=3746. Accessed September 22, 2005.

[3] New 2005 goals released: clinical alarm requirement cut from JCAHO priorities. Available at: aami.org/publications/AAMINews/2004/September/0904.jcaho.html. Accessed September 22, 2005.

[4] Chambrin MC. Alarms in the intensive care unit: how can the number of false alarms be reduced? Critical Care Forum 2001;5(4):184–8.

[5] Cropp AJ, Woods LA, Raney D, et al. Name that tone: the proliferation of alarms in the intensive care unit. Chest 1994;105(4):1217–20.

[6] Momhatan K, Hetu R, Tansley B. Audibility and identification of auditory alarms in the operating room and intensive care unit. Ergonomics 1993;36(10):1159–76.

[7] Finley GA, Cohen AJ. Perceived urgency of the anesthetist. Available at http://www.ahrq.gov/clinic/ptsafety/chap41b.htm. Accessed September 22, 2005.

[8] Mondor TA, Finley GA. The perceived urgency of auditory warning alarms used in the hospital operating room is inappropriate. Can J Anaesth 2003;50(3):221–8.

[9] Edworthy J, Hellier E. Fewer but better auditory alarms will improve patient safety. Quality Saf Health Care 2005;14:212–5.

[10] Clinical alarm management and integration: issues, changes, and emerging technologies, and clinical engineering initiatives. Available at: http://www.acce-htf.org/Clinical%20Alarms%20Management%20%20Integration.ppt. Accessed September 22, 2005.

[11] McIntosh N. Intensive care monitoring: past, present and future. Clin Med (Northfield Il) 2002;2(4):349–55.

[12] Schoenberg R, Sands DZ, Safran C. Making ICU alarms meaningful: a comparison of traditional vs trend based algorithm. Proceedings of American Medical Informatics Symposium, 1999, 379–83.

[13] Critical alarms and patient safety: ECRI's guide to developing effective alarm strategies and responding to JCAHO's alarm-safety goal. Health Devices 2002;31(11):397–417.

[14] Alarm enhancement systems for ventilators. Health Devices 2004;33(1):5–23.

[15] How and when do you test alarms? Briefings on Patient Safety 2003;12(4):4.

[16] Tsien CL, Fackler JC. Poor prognosis for existing monitors in the intensive care unit. Crit Care Med 1997;25(4):614–9.

[17] Keil O. Managing medical alarms: a practical approach to meeting the JCAHO national patient safety goal. Available at: www.clinicaldynamics.com/downloads/test_report_revB.pdf. Accessed 9.23.05.

[18] Richardson W. Home study program: clinical alarm systems testing—a program assessment model. AORN J 2004;80(2):280–93.

[19] Failure mode, effect, criticality analysis resources. Available at: www.jcaho.org/accredited+organizations/patient+safety/fmeca/fmeca+worksheets.htm. Accessed September 22, 2005.

[20] Physiologic monitoring systems. Health Devices 2005;34(1):5–45.

[21] Phillips J, Barnsteiner J. Clinical alarms: improving efficiency and effectiveness. Crit Care Nurs Q 2005;28:317–23.

ELSEVIER
SAUNDERS

Crit Care Nurs Clin N Am 18 (2006) 157–168

CRITICAL CARE
NURSING CLINICS
OF NORTH AMERICA

Practice Standards for ECG Monitoring in Hospital Settings: Executive Summary and Guide for Implementation

Barbara J. Drew, RN, PhD[a,*], Marjorie Funk, RN, PhD[b]

[a]School of Nursing, University of California, San Francisco, 2 Koret Way, San Francisco, CA 94143-0610, USA
[b]School of Nursing, Yale University, 100 Church Street South, P.O. Box 9740, New Haven, CT 06536-0740, USA

When hospital ECG monitoring was introduced more than 40 years ago, the goals were to track heart rate and detect arrhythmic cardiac arrest (ie, asystole or ventricular fibrillation). Today's goals encompass the diagnosis of complex arrhythmias (eg, differential diagnosis of wide QRS complex tachycardia), acute myocardial ischemia, and drug-induced prolonged QT interval. Although cardiac monitoring companies have provided many improvements, such as computer-assisted diagnosis of arrhythmias and ischemia, nursing oversight to interpret the significance of ECG events, based upon the individual patient's clinical situation, is critically important.

Recently, experts in the field of electrocardiology and cardiac monitoring convened to develop a practice standard for hospital ECG monitoring [1]. They called the document a standard, rather than a guideline, because their recommendations could not be based on evidence from large randomized clinical trials. Research to evaluate best practices for hospital ECG monitoring is almost nonexistent. Thus, the practice standard is based upon expert opinions regarding arrhythmia, ischemia, and QT interval monitoring. The practice standard can be downloaded from the American Heart Association's website [2]. Alternatively, the practice standard and a live video presentation that was filmed at the 2005 American Association of Critical-Care Nurses' National Teaching Institute can be obtained by searching for "Taste of NTI" at the AACN web site [3]. The live video presentation also displays the PowerPoint slides that were used in the presentation, which provides an excellent opportunity to show the 75-minute session at a hospital in-service seminar.

This executive summary reviews the high-priority elements of the practice standard, and covers practical aspects and frequently asked questions—not covered in the practice standard—that inevitably come up when clinicians try to implement them. The high-priority elements are the "class I" indications for arrhythmia, ischemia, and QT interval monitoring that are spelled out in the practice standard. Class I is defined as the clinical situations that have top priority for ECG monitoring. The reader is encouraged to refer to the longer practice standard to review class II (monitoring may be indicated) and class III (monitoring is unnecessary) categories. The reader also is referred to the practice standard for a detailed review/critique of the research literature that is available on the subject, and to obtain the extensive reference list that the experts used to support their recommendations.

Arrhythmia monitoring

Table 1 lists the clinical conditions that have top priority for arrhythmia monitoring with recommendations about how long monitoring should be maintained. These clinical conditions include all patients who are at significant risk for an immediate, life-threatening arrhythmia. If a patient is required to leave the monitored unit for diagnostic or therapeutic procedures, ECG monitoring should be continued with a portable monitor-defibrillator, and the patient

---

* Corresponding author.

E-mail address: barbara.drew@nursing.ucsf.edu (B.J. Drew).

Table 1
Recommendations for cardiac arrhythmia monitoring

Top priority for arrhythmia monitoring	Timeframe of monitoring
1. Patients resuscitated from cardiac arrest	1. Until cardioverter-defibrillator device implanted or reversible cause corrected (eg, hyperkalemia)
2. Patients in early phase of acute coronary syndromes (ST-elevation/non–ST-elevation MI, unstable angina), "rule-out" MI	2. Minimum 24 h for uncomplicated MI; until 24 hrs after complications resolved (eg, ongoing chest pain)
3. Patients with newly-diagnosed high-risk coronary lesions (eg, critical left main coronary artery stenosis)	3. Until intervention (e.g., revascularization)
4. Patients after cardiac surgery (record atrial electrogram from epicardial pacer wires with tachycardias of unknown origin)	4. Minimum 48–72 h; until hospital discharge in patients at risk for postoperative atrial fibrillation (eg, history of atrial fibrillation)
5. Patients after nonurgent percutaneous coronary intervention (angioplasty, stenting) with complications in catheterization laboratory (eg, vessel dissection, no reflow, suboptimal angiographic result)	5. Minimum 24 h; longer if arrhythmias or ischemia occur
6. Patients after implantation of automatic defibrillator or pacemaker lead who are pacemaker dependent (ie, unstable or absent rhythm without pacing)	6. 12–24 h after implantation
7. Patients with temporary or transcutaneous pacemaker	7. Until pacing no longer necessary and device removed or replaced with permanent device
8. Patients who have AV block: Wenkebach (unless stable long-term condition), Mobitz II, advanced (2:1 or higher), complete AV block, or new-onset bundle branch block in setting of acute MI	8. Until block resolves or definitive therapy (eg, permanent pacemaker)
9. Patients who have arrhythmias complicating WPW syndrome with rapid conduction over an accessory pathway (eg, atrial fibrillation with rate >150)	9. Until definitive therapy (usually catheter ablation)
10. Patients who have drug-induced long-QT syndrome	10. Until proarrhythmic drug discontinued and QT_C returned to predrug state and no QT-related arrhythmias
11. Patients who have intra-aortic balloon counterpulsation	11. Until weaned from intra-aortic balloon pump
12. Patients who have acute heart failure, pulmonary edema	12. Until signs/symptoms of acute heart failure resolved and no hemodynamically significant arrhythmias for 24 h
13. Patients who require intensive care (eg, major trauma, acute respiratory failure, sepsis, shock, pulmonary embolus, major noncardiac surgery, drug overdose)	13. Until weaned from mechanical ventilation and hemodynamically stable
14. Patients who undergo procedures that require conscious sedation or anesthesia	14. Until awake, alert, hemodynamically stable

Abbreviations: AV, atrioventricular; MI, myocardial infarction; WPW, Wolff-Parkinson-White.

should be accompanied by a health care provider who is skilled in ECG interpretation and defibrillation.

Nursing responsibilities in arrhythmia monitoring

When a patient is attached to an ECG monitor, a computer algorithm for arrhythmia detection is activated automatically; however, the computer algorithm is set to trigger an alarm when there is even a slight possibility of a life-threatening arrhythmia. Thus, a noisy signal that is due to the patient scratching an electrode or brushing his teeth may trigger an alarm that indicates ventricular tachycardia. Erroneous interpretation of such false alarms has resulted

in inappropriate treatment, including insertion of implantable devices [4]. For this reason, a major nursing responsibility is to distinguish true from false alarms.

Another responsibility in arrhythmia monitoring is to document the onset and termination of tachycardias because diagnostic clues to the arrhythmia mechanism may become evident at those times. To capture the termination of a tachycardia, the low alarm can be set 10 to 20 beats below the tachycardia rate so that a low alarm with accompanying rhythm strip is triggered when the patient converts to sinus rhythm. Setting an alarm to alert one at the time of tachycardia termination is especially prudent when administering ibutilide (Corvert) for the conversion of atrial fibrillation or flutter. Ibutilide is one of the drugs that can cause prolonged QT syndrome and the life-threatening arrhythmia, torsades de pointes. Torsades de pointes is a pause-dependent arrhythmia, which means it is triggered after a pause. Therefore, if torsades de pointes does occur after ibutilide administration, it will happen most likely at the time that atrial fibrillation or flutter converts to sinus rhythm when there is a pause. Thus, the monitor alarm can alert one at the time that defibrillation is most likely to be required.

A responsibility for nurses who care for patients after cardiac surgery is to document an atrial electrogram by recording a rhythm strip from atrial epicardial pacemaker wires whenever a patient develops a tachycardia of unknown mechanism [5]. During tachycardias, atrial activity often is not evident on the ECG tracing because P waves are buried within the rapidly occurring larger QRS-T waveforms. An atrial electrogram records larger atrial activity (P waves, flutter, or fibrillatory waves) than ventricular activity (QRS complexes), which often establishes the tachycardia mechanism and guides appropriate therapy. A simple way to record an immediate atrial electrogram from a bedside cardiac monitor is to put on rubber gloves, unsnap the chest (V) lead wire from the patient's chest, hold it against the tip of one of the atrial epicardial lead wires so metal is touching metal, and print a rhythm strip.

In most cases, however, patients in hospital monitored units who develop a tachycardia of unknown origin do not have atrial epicardial pacer wires available for recording. The next best way to determine tachycardia mechanism is to record a "stat" 12-lead ECG. Because tachycardias of clinical importance may be nonsustained, it is important to have standard 12-lead ECG carts readily available for immediate use, unless continuous 12-lead monitoring is being done.

ST-segment ischemia monitoring

In contrast to arrhythmia monitoring, ST-segment monitoring generally is not activated automatically when a patient is attached to a cardiac monitor. In addition, ST-segment software typically is provided as an option, rather than a required feature, so it is important to learn whether this capability exists in one's unit. It is not appropriate for all patients to be monitored for myocardial ischemia. For example, ischemia and infarction are rare in children, so ST-segment monitoring software is considered unnecessary in pediatric ICU monitors. Agitated patients whose ECG tracings are plagued with constant noise also are inappropriate for ST-segment monitoring. Activation of ST-segment monitoring is another source of false alarms that can be triggered in addition to those that are generated from the arrhythmia alarm system. Therefore, it is important not to evoke ischemia monitoring unless it is necessary, because of the "hassle" factor in sorting out multiple false alarms.

Table 2 lists the four clinical conditions that have top priority for ST-segment monitoring with recommendations about how long monitoring should be maintained. These clinical conditions include all patients who are at significant risk for myocardial ischemia which, if sustained, may result in the complication of acute myocardial infarction (MI) or re-MI after hospital admission. The authors of the practice standard point out that there have been no randomized clinical trials to determine whether ST-segment monitoring results in better patient outcomes. Therefore, the recommendations are based

Table 2
Recommendations for ST-segment ischemia monitoring

Top priority for ischemia monitoring	Timeframe of monitoring
1. Patients in early phase of acute coronary syndromes (ST-elevation/non–ST-elevation MI, unstable angina) or "rule-out" MI	1. Minimum 24 h and no ST events for 12–24 h
2. Patients who present to emergency department with chest pain/anginal equivalent	2. 8–12 h until negative biomarkers exclude acute MI
3. Patients after nonurgent percutaneous coronary intervention (angioplasty, stenting) with complications in catheterization laboratory (eg, vessel dissection, no reflow, or suboptimal angiographic result)	3. 24 h; longer if ST events occur
4. Patients who have possible variant angina due to coronary vasospasm	4. If diagnosis confirmed: until definitive therapy (eg, calcium-channel blocker) and no ST events for 12–24 h

upon the opinions of the expert group, several of whom have experienced the value of ischemia monitoring in individual cases.

Nursing responsibilities in ST-segment ischemia monitoring

After it has been determined that ischemia monitoring is warranted, it is important to select the individual patient's most sensitive ECG leads for detecting ischemia. The concept of monitoring a patient's "ST fingerprint" lead was introduced to assist in appropriate lead selection for patients who have acute MI or an ECG-documented ischemic episode [6]. Ischemic ST-T wave changes often are restricted to two or three ECG leads, depending upon the myocardial zone involved; the remaining leads show no abnormalities. The ST fingerprint lead is the one from a 12-lead ECG that shows the maximum ST segment deviation (either ST elevation or depression) during acute ischemia. In patients who had an acute MI, the best ECG to use to determine a patient's ST fingerprint lead usually is the first hospital ECG that was recorded in the emergency department before initiation of early reperfusion therapy. For patients who undergo angioplasty or stenting, a 12-lead ECG that was recorded during catheter balloon inflation provides the ST fingerprint pattern. Because these recordings require radiolucent electrodes and leads wires, they usually are made rarely unless a special protocol is set up in the cardiac catheterization laboratory. For patients who have unstable angina or other causes of transient myocardial ischemia, the 12-lead ECG that was documented during an anginal episode should be used to identify the ST fingerprint lead.

The ST fingerprint ECG pattern is unique to each patient (like an individual's fingerprint), and is dependent upon the location/extent of the patient's coronary artery disease. Selecting the patient's ST fingerprint lead is the best way to detect subsequent ischemic events in an individual patient. For example, if the maximal ST-segment deviation in a patient who has an acute anterior wall MI is lead V_3, this lead is most sensitive to confirm successful reperfusion therapy (ie, rapidly resolving ST elevation) or to detect coronary artery reocclusion following the reperfusion therapy.

To detect abrupt reocclusion following percutaneous coronary interventions, such as angioplasty or stenting when no 12-lead ECGs have been recorded during catheter balloon inflation, knowing the intervention artery provides guidance for appropriate lead selection [7–9]. Research has shown that leads III, aVF, and II (in order of maximal to least ST elevation) are the most sensitive ECG leads to detect occlusion of the right coronary artery. Although the routinely monitored lead II typically has the least ST elevation among these three "inferior" leads, it has the advantage of having the most prominent R wave in most individuals (ie, greatest signal-to-noise ratio), which provides the cleanest tracing for accurate heart rate detection. Lead V_2 or V_3 is the most sensitive lead to detect occlusion of the left anterior descending coronary artery. Occlusion of the left circumflex artery is most difficult to detect because it produces ischemia of the posterior left ventricular wall, which is the furthest away from anterior precordial electrode sites. Lead V_3 is considered the best of the 12 standard leads to detect occlusion of the left circumflex artery, because it usually has the greatest reciprocal ST segment depression compared with other leads.

After determining the appropriate ECG lead, ST alarm parameters need to be set above and below the patient's baseline ST level. Most patients who are hospitalized in monitored units do not have normal, isoelectric ST segments, even during times when they are not experiencing ischemia [10]. These ST deviations may be due to digitalis therapy, left ventricular hypertrophy, bundle branch block, or other nonischemic conditions. The practice standard recommends that alarm parameters be set 1 mm above and below the baseline ST level in patients who are at high risk for ischemia and at 2 mm for more stable patients [1].

As with arrhythmia monitoring, nursing oversight is required to distinguish true from false ST alarms. The most common cause of false ST alarms is a change of ST amplitude that is due to a change in the patient's body position (eg, turning from a supine to a left-side-lying position) [11]. A clue to a false alarm that is due to body position change is a change in the size or direction of the QRS complex that accompanies the ST segment change [12]. A true ischemic ST event is not expected to cause a change in QRS morphology. The practice standard recommends the following: (1) when an ST alarm sounds and a patient is found in a side-lying position, the patient should be returned to the supine position. (2) If the ST segment deviation disappears (ie, returns to the baseline level), it should be considered a false alarm. If in doubt, the patient can be turned again to the side-lying position to confirm that the ECG changes are related to body position changes.

Other nursing responsibilities include a careful skin preparation and consistent electrode placement. If an electrode requires relocation because of skin

Table 3
QT-prolonging drugs

Generic name	Brand name(s)	Clinical use
Amiodarone	Cordarone, Pacerone	Antiarrhythmic
Arsenic trioxide	Trisenox	Cancer/leukemia
Bepridil	Vascor	Antianginal
Chlorpromazine	Thorazine	Antipsychotic
Cisapride	Propulsid	GI stimulant
Clarithromycin	Biaxin	Antibiotic
Disopyramide	Norpace	Antiarrhythmic
Dofetilide	Tikosyn	Antiarrhythmic
Domperidone	Motilium	Antiemetic
Droperidol	Inapsine	Sedative; antiemetic
Erythromycin	E.E.S., Erythrocin	Antibiotic
Halofantrine	Halfan	Antimalarial
Haloperidol	Haldol	Antipsychotic
Ibutilide	Corvert	Antiarrhythmic
Levomethadyl	Orlaam	Opiate agonist
Mesoridazine	Serentil	Antipsychotic
Methadone	Dolophine, Methadose	Opiate agonist
Pentamidine	NebuPent, Pentam	Anti-infective
Pimozide	Orap	Antipsychotic
Procainamide	Pronestyl, Procanbid	Antiarrhythmic
Quinidine	Quinaglute, Cardioquin, Quinidex Extentabs	Antiarrhythmic
Sotalol	Betapace	Antiarrhythmic
Sparfloxacin	Zagam	Antibiotic
Thioridazine	Mellaril	Antipsychotic

Drugs in bold require ECG monitoring; others require monitoring if patient has risk (eg, >1 drug).
Abbreviation: GI, gastrointestinal.

irritation or placement of a defibrillator pad, documentation of a rhythm strip before and after the electrodes have been moved will explain resultant ST trend changes that may otherwise be misinterpreted as ischemia. Although graphic displays of ST trend data may be helpful to identify potential ischemic events, they are no substitute for documentation of the actual ECG waveforms. For example, any arrhythmia that is associated with secondary ST-T wave abnormalities (eg, ventricular rhythms or new bundle branch block) will cause changes that mimic ischemia on the ST graphic trends.

Monitoring for prolonged QT interval and proarrhythmia

The QT interval is measured from the onset of the QRS complex to the end of the T wave, and it approximates the time that it takes the ventricles to repolarize. Certain drugs and conditions can cause abnormally long repolarization times, which places the patient at risk for developing the malignant ventricular arrhythmia, torsades de pointes. The QT-prolonging drugs are listed in Table 3, and can be found on the web site that is maintained by the University of Arizona [13]. The six antiarrhythmic drugs that are shown in bold in Table 3 are especially likely to cause proarrhythmia; their initiation requires ECG monitoring. Polypharmacy with QT-prolonging drugs also makes a patient more likely to develop proarrhythmia (Table 4). For example, if a patient takes methadone for drug abuse, initiation of erythromycin poses more of a risk for torsades de pointes than if the patient were on erythromycin alone.

Table 4
Recommendations for QT interval monitoring for detection of proarrhythmia

Top priority for QT monitoring	Timeframe of monitoring
1. Patients started on antiarrhythmic drug known to cause torsades de pointes (especially, disopyramide, dofetilide, ibutilide, procainamide, quinidine, sotalol)	1. Until drug is discontinued or dosage stable and no prolonged QT_C (>0.48 s, women; >0.47 s, men) and no QT-related arrhythmias (polymorphic ventricular ectopy, couplets, nonsustained VT, torsades de pointes)
2. Patients who overdose from potentially proarrhythmic agent	2. Until drug levels decreased and no QT-related arrhythmias
3. Patients who have new-onset bradyarrhythmias (eg, complete heart block, long sinus pauses)	3. Until bradyarrhythmia resolved or definitive therapy (eg, permanent pacemaker)
4. Patients who have severe hypokalemia or hypomagnesemia	4. Until electrolyte disorder corrected and no QT-related arrhythmias

Abbreviation: VT, ventricular tachycardia.

Amiodarone causes extreme prolongation of the QT interval, but it is not featured in bold type in Table 3 as a high-risk drug. The underlying cellular mechanism that produces torsades de pointes is an unequal repolarization response to a drug by epicardial, midmyocardial, and endocardial layers of the ventricular wall. Unlike drugs that have a high risk for proarrhythmia, amiodarone prolongs repolarization time in all three myocardial layers equally. Thus, the heterogeneity of repolarization that is required for development of torsades de pointes is not present. Electrolyte disorders (especially hypokalemia or hypomagnesemia), severe bradycardias (especially complete heart block or long sinus pauses, including at the time of tachycardia termination), and acute neurologic events (especially subarachnoid hemorrhage) are other conditions that can cause prolonged QT and torsades de pointes.

Because the QT interval normally gets longer with slower heart rates and shorter with faster heart rates, the QT interval must be corrected for heart rate (QT_C) when assessing whether a patient is developing dangerous QT prolongation over time. No commercially available cardiac monitor provides for automatic measurement, trending, and alarms for QT interval assessment. Fortunately, QT measurement does not have to be monitored continuously, because QT prolongation does not develop instantaneously, as do cardiac arrhythmias and ischemia. Several cardiac monitoring companies provide computed-assisted electronic calipers to measure QT and RR intervals, from which the QT_C can be calculated by the monitor. The use of electronic calipers requires the nurse to determine the onset of the QRS complex and the end of the T wave. For this reason, it is ideal if the cardiac monitoring system allows one to increase the size of waveforms (from standardization of 1 to 2, 3, or 4) and to increase the recording speed (from 25 mm/s to 50 mm/s). Such manipulation produces large, stretched out QRS–T waveforms, which makes it easy to be accurate in marking the measurement points.

If electronic calipers are unavailable, manual calculation of QT_C is required. The most common QT correction formula that is used in clinical practice was introduced by Bazett [14]: QT_C = QT interval divided by the square root of the R-R interval measured in seconds. Because this formula requires a calculator, which may discourage its use, nurses should evaluate QT measurement features of various cardiac monitoring brands when it is time to purchase new equipment.

A reasonable recommendation (in the absence of adequate research) is to document the QT_C interval before (baseline interval) and at least every 8 to 12 hours after the initiation, increased dosage, or overdosage of QT-prolonging drugs. If QT_C prolongation is observed, more frequent measurements should be documented. A QT_C is considered prolonged if it exceeds 0.47 second in men and 0.48 second in women. A QT_C of greater than 0.50 second is considered dangerous prolongation in men and women. When the QT_C reaches this point, the physician or nurse practitioner should be notified to discontinue the drug, especially if QT-related arrhythmias are present. An ECG lead with a well-defined T wave should be chosen for measuring QT intervals. Moreover, the same ECG lead should be used to make serial measurements in a given patient so that an increase in the QT interval represents increased ventricular repolarization, rather than changes in waveform morphology between various ECG leads.

How long QT_C measurement should be continued depends upon the drug half-life, how long it takes for the drug to be eliminated from the body (which may depend on renal function), whether the drug is given once or as an ongoing therapy, how long it takes for the QT_C to return to the predrug baseline, and whether the ECG shows QT-related arrhythmias. For example, the drug ibutilide, which is administered as a one-time treatment for termination of atrial fibrillation or flutter, has not been reported to produce torsades de pointes after 4 hours of administration. Thus, it is unnecessary to monitor QT_C after 4 hours in patients who receive this drug.

The ECG signs of impending torsades de pointes include one or more of the following: (1) QT_C is more than 0.50 second, (2) frequent polymorphic ventricular ectopy and couplets, (3) T wave alternans (alternation of T wave size with every other beat), (4) prominent U waves (>1 mm) that may be fused with the T wave and resemble a camel's hump, or (5) nonsustained polymorphic ventricular tachycardia that is initiated on the T wave of a beat following a pause (usually the beat after a compensatory pause following a ventricular premature beat). If these ECG signs occur, torsades de pointes is highly likely to occur and defibrillation should be immediately available. Patients should not be transported off the unit for diagnostic or therapeutic procedures, and they should be in a unit with the highest possible ECG monitoring surveillance. The culprit drug must be discontinued immediately and hypokalemia, if present, should be corrected because it makes triggering of torsades de pointes more likely. In addition, magnesium should be administered regardless of the serum magnesium level because it is believed to stabilize cardiac membranes.

Cardiac monitoring lead systems

It is beyond the scope of this executive summary to describe the plethora of ECG lead configurations that are available with the current generation of cardiac monitors. A detailed description of each lead configuration with corresponding figures that illustrate accurate electrode placement is provided in the practice standard [1]. Instead, this discussion focuses on answers to common questions that arise in clinical practice.

Where should limb leads be placed for recording a 12-lead ECG?

To record a resting 12-lead ECG using a standard ECG cart, the right arm (RA) and left arm (LA) leads should be placed on the corresponding wrists or forearms, and the right leg (RL) and left leg (LL) leads should be placed on the corresponding ankles or skin over the tibia. All diagnoses that require precise measurement of the amplitude (size or height) of waveforms are based on research using such wrist/ankle limb lead locations. Therefore, to make diagnoses, such as atrial enlargement or ventricular hypertrophy, this standard lead placement is important. Often, this type of 12-lead ECG is called a "diagnostic ECG" because all amplitude criteria can be used for all possible ECG diagnoses.

In hospitals with an ECG storage system, it is assumed that no modification of standard lead placement has been used. If ECGs are stored with limb leads placed on the torso, there may be slight differences in waveforms (especially in the six limb leads), which may be misleading when comparisons are made of serial ECGs. For example, most 12-lead ECG carts have sophisticated computer interpretation algorithms that compare the current ECG with a previously stored ECG. If a different limb lead placement is used between the current and previously stored ECG, the computer interpretation may indicate that there has been a change in QRS axis or that there are changes in T wave morphology that may be suggestive of myocardial ischemia.

When limb leads are moved from the wrists and ankles to the upper arms or thighs, there is only a slight, if any, change in the waveforms. Such alternate limb lead placement probably is acceptable for recording a diagnostic standard 12-lead ECG; however, placement of electrodes over large muscle groups (deltoids, quadriceps) may create a noisy signal. The closer to the heart from the wrists/ankles that the limb leads are moved, the greater is the potential for waveform change, which threatens the

validity of serial comparisons. It should also be pointed out that the RL electrode does not contribute to the waveform morphology; therefore, it can be placed anywhere on the body. For example, during procedures that use the right groin area to insert catheters, the RL electrode can be placed next to the LL electrode without a change in the ECG tracing.

When a patient is monitored continuously with a 12-lead ECG (eg, for exercise testing or bedside monitoring), it is impractical to place limb leads on the wrists and ankles, because it tethers the patient and creates an unacceptably noisy signal with limb movement that creates numerous false alarms. For this reason, the limb leads are placed on the torso. The RA and LA electrodes should be placed just below the clavicle and as close as possible to the shoulder. RL and LL electrodes should be placed on the right and left abdomen below the rib cage. Using this placement, the 12-lead ECG is similar, but not identical, to the standard 12-lead ECG. If arm electrodes are moved medially toward the sternum, more striking changes in waveforms occur, which make the resultant 12-lead ECG invalid. RA and LA electrodes can be placed high on the patient's upper back as long as they are close to the respective shoulders. This alternate placement may be desired to protect a future pacemaker site, which often is below the clavicle. Electrodes that are left in place for long periods of time can produce skin rashes or irritation, which may compromise future surgical sites and can lead to postoperative infection [15].

It is important to emphasize that when a torso-positioned 12-lead ECG that is obtained from cardiac monitoring equipment differs in waveform morphology from the ECG that was recorded with a standard ECG cart, it should not be substituted for the periodic "diagnostic" ECGs that are ordered for the patient. If, however, no discernable differences exist between the cardiac monitor and ECG-cart tracings, the 12-lead ECG that was obtained from the monitor probably can serve as a substitute if it was recorded with the patient in a supine position.

Are derived 12-lead ECGs comparable to standard 12-lead ECGs in diagnostic accuracy?

Many diagnoses that require a diagnostic 12-lead ECG are unimportant to detect while a patient is being monitored in a hospital unit. For example, the diagnoses of atrial enlargement or ventricular hypertrophy are unimportant to detect because they do not require intervention in an immediate care setting. Moreover, many diagnoses that are of consequence during cardiac monitoring can be diagnosed accurately with a single ECG lead. For example, atrial fibrillation and atrioventricular (AV) block can be diagnosed readily by observing a single lead rhythm strip; however, two clinically important diagnoses, differentiation of wide QRS tachycardias and detection of acute myocardial ischemia, require multiple leads for accurate interpretation. To distinguish ventricular tachycardia from supraventricular tachycardia with a wide QRS complex that is due to bundle branch block or aberrant ventricular conduction, one needs to look for criteria in the limb leads (QRS axis) and the precordial leads (QRS morphology in $V_{1,}$, V_2, and V_6) [16]. Likewise, to detect ischemia in multiple zones of the heart, one needs to look for ST segment changes in the limb leads (inferior wall of the heart; ie, leads II, III, aVF) and the precordial leads (anterior wall of the heart). These two clinically relevant diagnoses can also be episodic and last just minutes (eg, nonsustained ventricular tachycardia or an anginal ischemic episode). As a result, clinicians frequently do not have time to capture these important events by recording a standard 12-lead ECG.

One strategy for documenting wide QRS tachycardias and myocardial ischemia with multiple leads is to monitor all 12 ECG leads continuously. Several cardiac monitoring companies provide for 12-lead ECG monitoring; however, the 10 electrodes and lead wires are cumbersome and difficult to maintain, and may get in the way of surgical wounds, defibrillator pads, and the recording of echocardiograms and chest radiographs. The six precordial leads are especially difficult to maintain, because of chest hair in men and breast tissue in women. For this reason, "reduced lead set" technology was developed. Reduced lead set technology derives 12 ECG leads from a small number of leads/electrodes. The EASI system (Philips, Andover, Massachusetts), which requires just five electrodes, was the first derived 12-lead ECG to be introduced in cardiac monitors. The EASI 12-lead is comparable to the standard ECG for detection of acute myocardial ischemia [17–19] and diagnosis of wide QRS tachycardias [20]. No reduced lead set ECG is identical to the standard ECG, and it should not be compared with previously recorded standard ECGs for diagnoses that require serial ECG assessment. For example, if a 12-lead ECG that was recorded using a standard ECG cart in the emergency department shows normal, upright T waves, and the derived 12-lead ECG that was recorded from the bedside monitor 30 minutes later shows T wave inversion, one cannot conclude that the patient developed new T wave abnormalities of ischemia. As is the case for any 12-lead ECG that is derived from a reduced number of electrodes/leads, serial ECG

comparisons should be made using the same recording technique.

What are the best landmarks to use in placing precordial leads? Should they be placed on top or underneath breasts in women?

The single most important landmark for accurate precordial lead placement is the sternal angle (also referred to as the Angle of Louis). This bony prominence in the upper sternum is caused by fusion of the upper and lower sternum in utero. The sternal angle marks the point where the second rib joins the sternum. The best way to find this landmark is as follows. With the patient recumbent, the suprasternal notch at the base of the throat is located. Just below this notch is the flat part of the upper sternum, which is called the manubrium. When placing the index and middle fingers together with fingertips pointing laterally, the sternal angle can be felt just below these two fingers. The fingers are next moved up over the bony prominence of the sternal angle to just below it. Next, the fingers are moved to the right side of the sternum, which corresponds to the second intercostal space. From the second intercostal space, it is easy to palpate down to the third and fourth intercostal spaces. Lead V_1 is placed in the fourth intercostal space at the right sternal border. This lead is often called the "anchor" lead, because all other precordial leads are placed in relation to it. If lead V_1 is misplaced, all of the precordial leads probably will be inaccurate.

Clinicians often ask why one does not palpate down from the clavicle to the first intercostal space. The answer is that some individuals have a palpable first intercostal space, whereas others do not; therefore, the method described above is a better strategy for locating the fourth intercostal space. In patients who have had sternotomy incisions, the sternum may not have knit together seamlessly, and locating the sternal angle may be difficult; however, one can locate the suprasternal notch and approximate the length of the manubrium with two fingers to determine where the sternal angle would be expected to be.

In elderly women with pendulous breasts, chest electrodes should be placed under, rather than on top of, the breast unless the fifth intercostal space (for V_{4-6}) is clearly above the breast. Pendulous breasts in elderly women attach to the chest wall at the same place as in younger women. Thus, if the tip of the breast is lifted up, an electrode can be placed on the chest wall just below where the breast attaches. The consequence of placing precordial leads on top of the breast is that the height of precordial R waves may be smaller because of the greater distance between the electrode and the heart. This may be interpreted as "loss of R wave voltage that is suggestive of anterior MI." In addition, placing electrodes on top of the breast may create baseline wander on the ECG from movement of breast tissue.

What precordial leads are misplaced most often in textbook diagrams and educational materials that are provided with ECG machines and monitoring equipment?

Most often, leads V_5 and V_6 are shown as following the fifth intercostal space laterally, which curves superiorly from the V_4 midclavicular line. The proper position for leads V_5 and V_6 is at the same horizontal level as V_4, which means that they often fall on or below the sixth rib.

What type of skin preparation helps to minimize a noisy signal and false alarms?

Carefully preparing the skin by cleaning the electrode sites with soap and water and drying with a rough washcloth or gauze is worth the extra minutes, because of the time that is saved in responding to false alarms. If the patient is diaphoretic or the skin excessively oily, an alcohol pad may be used, but this may dehydrate and cause increased skin resistance. Excessive hair at electrode sites should be clipped rather than shaved because shaving may cause nicking and irritation.

Are dedicated monitor watchers necessary?

Research that was published in 1997 showed that a dedicated nurse monitor watcher was associated with greater accuracy in the detection of clinically important arrhythmias [21] and a reduced incidence of sustained ventricular tachycardia [22]. Dedicated monitor watchers are appropriate on units where surveillance of arrhythmias, ischemia, and QT prolongation is a high priority, and monitors cannot be observed continually by nurses because of their direct care responsibilities.

Qualifications of staff required to provide safe and effective oversight in the interpretation of ECG monitoring data

Cardiac monitoring is performed in a wide variety of hospital units, including adult and pediatric criti-

---

Box 1. Specific ECG abnormalities

Normal rhythms
  Sinus rhythm, sinus bradycardia, sinus arrhythmia, sinus tachycardia
Intraventricular conduction defects
  Right and left bundle branch block, aberrant ventricular conduction
Bradyarrhythmias
  Inappropriate sinus bradycardia, sinus node pause/arrest, nonconducted atrial premature beats, junctional rhythm, AV blocks (first degree, second degree [Wenckebach, Mobitz II], advanced [$\geq$2:1], third degree [complete heart block]), asystole, pulseless electrical activity, sino-ventricular rhythm (severe hyperkalemia)
Tachyarrhythmias
  Supraventricular
    Paroxysmal supraventricular tachycardia (AV nodal reentrant, AV reentrant), atrial fibrillation, atrial flutter, multifocal atrial tachycardia, atrial tachycardia with and without 2:1 block, accelerated junctional rhythm
  Ventricular
    Accelerated ventricular rhythm, nonsustained and sustained monomorphic ventricular tachycardia, nonsustained and sustained polymorphic ventricular tachycardia, prolonged QT interval–associated ventricular ectopy and torsades de pointes, ventricular fibrillation
Premature beats
  Supraventricular (atrial, junctional), ventricular
Pacemaker electrocardiography
  Failure to capture, failure to pace (no pacer output), failure to sense, failure to capture both ventricles in biventricular pacing
ECG abnormalities of acute myocardial ischemia
  Criteria for ischemia for ST segment elevation, depression, and T wave inversion
Muscle or other artifacts simulating arrhythmias

cal care units, progressive care units, emergency departments, high-risk obstetrics, cardiac catheterization and electrophysiology laboratories, operating rooms, and postanesthesia recovery units. Each unit has different goals for monitoring. For example, in emergency departments, ST-segment ischemia monitoring is important so patients who have acute coronary

---

Box 2. General electrophysiologic concepts

Automaticity
  Physiologic pacemakers,
    overdrive suppression
Excitation
  Refractory periods
Conduction
  Conduction velocity, concealed
    conduction, anterograde and
    retrograde conduction
Sinus node physiology
  Normal ranges of sinus rate with age,
    effects of autonomic tone (vaso-
    vagal reactions, resting/sleep,
    activity/exercise), effects of drugs
AV node physiology
  Effects of atrial rate, autonomic tone,
    (resting/sleep, activity/exercise),
    and drugs
Wide versus narrow QRS complexes
QT/U intervals
  Relation to rate, gender differences,
    drugs that require QT_C
    assessment, pause dependency
Classification of arrhythmias
  Sustained versus nonsustained,
    monomorphic versus polymorphic,
    symptomatic versus asymptomatic
Hemodynamic effects of arrhythmias
  Influence of rate, heart disease,
    atrioventricular synchrony, left
    ventricular synchrony
Implantable devices
  Function of pacemakers (including
    biventricular pacemakers),
    automatic defibrillators
Acute myocardial ischemia
  ST elevation MI (anterior, inferior,
    right ventricular; ST recovery in-
    dicative of successful reperfusion;
    reperfusion arrhythmias; intermit-
    tent reperfusion; ECG leads that
    reflect occlusion of three main
    coronary arteries)
  Non-ST elevation MI
  Transient myocardial ischemia
    (effects of body position changes
    mimicking ischemia)
Syncope
Effects of common antiarrhythmic drugs,
  rate control versus rhythm control

Box 3. Specific monitoring skills

Operation of monitoring system
  (arrhythmia, ST segment monitoring)
Recognition of limitations of computer
  algorithms (ability to identify
  false alarms)
Proper skin preparation for
  applying electrodes
Accurate electrode placement and lead
  wire connection
Appropriate setting of heart rate and
  ST alarm parameters
Recording of standard 12-lead ECG
  (landmarks for accurate
  lead placement)
Measurement of heart rate
Measurement of intervals (PR, QRS,
  QT, RR, QT_C,), use of ECG calipers
Recognition of atrial activity
Evaluation of pauses
Diagnosis of common (eg, atrial
  fibrillation) and hemodynamically
  significant (eg, ventricular
  tachycardia) arrhythmias
Recording from postoperative
  epicardial pacer wires
  (including electrical safety)
Ability to intervene (unit protocols for
  responding to, reporting,
  and documenting)
  Defibrillation/cardioversion
  The patient who has bradycardia
  The patient who has tachycardia
  The patient who has syncope
  The patient who has
    cardiorespiratory arrest
  The patient with an implanted
    device (new or chronic)
  The patient with a temporary
    transvenous pacemaker
  The patient with a
    transcutaneous pacemaker

syndromes will not be sent home mistakenly. Medical and nursing leadership in each hospital unit with cardiac monitoring should determine the staff proficiencies required to monitor patients safely and effectively, given the types of patients that are cared for in a particular unit.

In units that treat a high proportion of cardiac patients where ECG monitoring is a high priority, nursing staff should understand specific ECG abnormalities (Box 1) and general electrophysiologic concepts (Box 2), and be proficient in monitoring skills (Box 3). Nurses who are responsible for ECG monitoring in any hospital unit should receive formal orientation and training that is specific to the type of monitoring system that is being used and the anticipated goals of monitoring for patients in the unit. Appropriate training must include didactic content and "hands-on" practice with return demonstration. Demonstration of accurate electrode placement is especially important because inaccurate electrode placement is common in hospital units [23], and can result in misdiagnosis. With input from key physicians who treat patients in a given unit, training should include what ECG events should be reported to physicians and when "stat" 12-lead ECGs should be recorded.

To ensure ongoing safe and effective ECG monitoring and to determine the need for refresher courses, a quality improvement program should be initiated. Measures of quality might include a review of all cardiac arrests in the unit (eg, time to first shock for life-threatening arrhythmias), the diagnostic accuracy of rhythm interpretations, appropriateness and quality of 12-lead ECGs recorded in response to detected rhythms or cardiac symptoms (eg, chest pain), the timeliness of human review of computer-generated alarms and rhythm strips, and the incorporation of clinically significant rhythm strips (eg, tachycardia onset and termination) into the permanent medical record. Measures of quality also would include documentation of QT_C measurements in patients who are started on QT-prolonging drugs, and activation of ST-segment ischemia monitoring in patients who have acute coronary syndromes. Additionally, there should be periodic audits of electrode placement.

Summary

Important clinical decisions, such as a patient's need for drug therapy, further diagnostic testing, cardiology consultation, transfer back to an ICU, extension of hospitalization, and more, are made every day using ECG monitoring data. Published reports of misdiagnosis of ECG monitoring data indicate that adverse patient outcomes may result from undertreatment or the wrong therapy. The expert writing group developed the practice standard that is summarized in this document to improve the safety and effectiveness of hospital ECG monitoring, and in so doing, to improve patient care and outcomes. The responsibility for incorporating the practice standards in hospital units ultimately rests on the shoulders of nursing staff who attach patients to cardiac monitors and observe their ECG rhythms.

References

[1] Drew BJ, Califf RM, Funk M, et al. Practice standards for electrocardiographic monitoring in hospital settings. Circulation 2004;110:2721–46.
[2] American Heart Association. Available at: http://www.americanheart.org.
[3] Available at: http://www.AACN.org.
[4] Knight BP, Pelosi F, Michaud GF, et al. Clinical consequences of electrocardiographic artifact mimicking ventricular tachycardia. New Engl J Med 1999;341:1270–4.
[5] Waldo AL, MacLean WAH, Cooper TB, et al. The use of temporarily placed epicardial wire electrodes for the diagnosis and treatment of cardiac arrhythmias following open heart surgery. J Thorac Cardiovasc Surg 1987;76:500–5.
[6] Krucoff MW, Parente AR, Bottner RK, et al. Stability of multilead ST segment "fingerprints" over time after percutaneous transluminal coronary angioplasty and its usefulness in detecting reocclusion. Am J Cardiol 1988;61:1232–7.
[7] Aldrich HR, Hindman NB, Hinohara T, et al. Identification of the optimal electrocardiographic leads for detecting acute epicardial injury in acute myocardial infarction. Am J Cardiol 1987;59:20–3.
[8] Bush HS, Ferguson JJ, Angelini P, et al. Twelve-lead electrocardiographic evaluation of ischemia during percutaneous transluminal coronary angioplasty and its correlation with acute reocclusion. Am Heart J 1991;121:1591–9.
[9] Drew BJ, Tisdale LA. ST segment monitoring for coronary artery reocclusion following thrombolytic therapy and coronary angioplasty: identification of optimal bedside monitoring leads. Am J Crit Care 1993;2:280–92.
[10] Drew BJ, Wung SF, Adams MG, et al. Bedside diagnosis of myocardial ischemia with ST-segment monitoring technology: measurement issues for real-time clinical decision-making and trial designs. J Electrocardiol 1998;30:157–65.
[11] Drew BJ, Adams MG. Clinical consequences of ST-segment changes caused by body position mimicking

transient myocardial ischemia: hazards of ST-segment monitoring? J Electrocardiol 2001;34:261–4.

[12] Feldman T, Borow K, Neumann A, et al. Relation of electrocardiographic R wave amplitude to changes in left ventricular chamber size and position in normal subjects. Am J Cardiol 1985;55:1168–74.

[13] www.torsades.org.

[14] Bazett HC. An analysis of the time-relations of electrocardiograms. Heart 1920;7:353–62.

[15] Shalaby A, Squier C, Muder R. An intervention to halt surgical site infections in implantable cardio-verter defibrillator recipients. Heart Rhythm (Suppl) 2004;1:S175.

[16] Drew BJ, Scheinman MM. ECG criteria to distinguish between aberrantly-conducted supraventricular tachy-cardia and ventricular tachycardia: practical aspects for the immediate care setting. Pacing Clin Electrophysiol 1995;18:2194–208.

[17] Drew BJ, Adams MG, Pelter MM, et al. ST segment monitoring with a derived 12-lead electrocardiogram is superior to routine CCU monitoring. Am J Crit Care 1996;5:198–206.

[18] Drew BJ, Adams MG, Pelter MM, et al. Comparison of standard and derived 12-lead electrocardiograms for diagnosis of coronary angioplasty-induced myocardial ischemia. Am J Cardiol 1997;79:639–44.

[19] Drew BJ, Pelter MM, Wung SF, et al. Accuracy of the EASI 12-lead electrocardiogram compared to the standard 12-lead electrocardiogram for diagnosing multiple cardiac abnormalities. J Electrocardiol 1999;32(Suppl):38–47.

[20] Drew BJ, Scheinman MM, Evans GT. Comparison of a vectorcardiographically derived 12-lead electro-cardiogram with the conventional electrocardiogram during wide QRS complex tachycardia, and its poten-tial application for continuous bedside monitoring. Am J Cardiol 1992;69:612–8.

[21] Stukshis I, Funk M, Johnson CR, Parkosewich JA. Accuracy of detection of clinically important dysrhyth-mias with and without a dedicated monitor watcher. Am J Crit Care 1997;6:312–7.

[22] Funk M, Parkosewich JA, Johnson CR, et al. Effect of dedicated monitor watchers on patient outcomes. Am J Crit Care 1997;6:318–23.

[23] Drew BJ, Ide B, Sparacino PSA. Accuracy of bedside electrocardiographic monitoring: a report on current practices of critical care nurses. Heart Lung 1991;20:597–609.

ELSEVIER
SAUNDERS

Crit Care Nurs Clin N Am 18 (2006) 169 – 177

CRITICAL CARE
NURSING CLINICS
OF NORTH AMERICA

Continuous ST-Segment Monitoring: Raising the Bar

Sonya A. Flanders, RN, BSN, CCRN

Baylor University Medical Center, 3500 Gaston Avenue, Dallas, TX 75246, USA

Recent publications strongly advocate for the clinical use of continuous ST-segment monitoring to aid in the earliest possible detection of myocardial ischemia [1–3]. Nonetheless, there is still a gap between these recommendations and clinical practice. Only about 50% of critical care units reported the use of routine monitoring of ST-segments in a national survey that was conducted by Patton and Funk [4]. Furthermore, the use of this technology outside of the critical care arena is unknown. Colleagues from across the United States indicate that ST-segments are not a routine electrocardiogram (ECG) parameter that is monitored continuously, despite the expert recommendations to do so and research that links ST-segment monitoring to improved patient outcomes. This article reviews the clinical value of continuous ST-segment monitoring and practice recommendations, and explores strategies for implementation.

The value of ST-segment monitoring

Traditionally, the 12-lead ECG has been the principal tool for identification of ECG changes that are associated with myocardial ischemia, injury, and infarction. One limitation of this technique is the static nature of the 12-lead ECG, which captures only 10 seconds of ECG data. Clinicians often obtain the 12-lead ECG when the patient complains of symptoms that are suggestive of myocardial ischemia. Because 80% to 90% of ischemic episodes are known to be clinically silent, most events are likely to be missed by a conventional 12-lead ECG [1,6]. Patients who complain of atypical symptoms, such as short-

ness of breath or indigestion, also may be overlooked. Almost 2 decades ago Krucoff and colleagues [5] described the monitoring of ST "fingerprints" as being useful for the detection of coronary reocclusion following percutaneous transluminal coronary angioplasty. The ST fingerprint is described as the patient's unique, reproducible pattern of ST-segment deviations in relation to anatomy of the occluded coronary artery [1]. Because the ST fingerprint varies among individuals, the more leads that can be monitored simultaneously, the greater is the likelihood that transient ischemic events will be detected. Whenever possible, all 12 ECG leads should be monitored continuously for ST-segment changes.

Plentiful research is available to support ST-segment monitoring. Fesmire and colleagues [7] conducted a study in the emergency department setting to determine the value of monitoring a patient with an initial 12-lead ECG versus automated serial ECG monitoring, which included automated sampling of ST-segments every 20 seconds. The study included 1000 adult patients who presented to the emergency department with chest pain suspicious for coronary ischemia. The researchers concluded that serial ECGs with ST-sampling showed significantly greater sensitivity for the detection of acute ischemic coronary events.

Other studies have been conducted in a variety of clinical circumstances, in which ST-segment pattern analysis was correlated with patient outcomes and supported its value as a prognostic indicator [8]. In an analysis of 237 cardiac patients on a telemetry unit who had ST-segment monitoring by way of continuous 12-lead ECG, those who experienced transient myocardial ischemia were more than eight times more likely to have complications in the hospital [9]. Patel and colleagues [10] also studied the prognostic

---

E-mail address: sonyaf@baylorhealth.edu

value of continuous ST-segment monitoring. Using an observational study technique, 212 patients who had unstable angina, but no acute myocardial infarction (MI), received standardized medical treatment and had their ST-segments monitored continuously for 48 hours. Fifteen percent of the patients experienced a total of 132 episodes of ischemia, 104 of which were clinically silent. Of all of the factors that were analyzed, transient myocardial ischemia was the most important predictor of adverse prognosis, including death, MI, and emergent revascularization. It follows that, through the use of continuous ST-segment monitoring, ischemic episodes that previously may have been missed could be identified, and such episodes that require reperfusion strategies could be treated more rapidly. Earlier treatment often allows myocardial preservation, which has a positive impact on mortality and morbidity. At this time, ECG monitoring is the single most practical method for the ongoing observation and detection of ischemic events [1]. Although many patients who undergo ST-segment monitoring may never experience an acute ischemic event, every patient deserves the benefit that this technology can provide, should such an event occur.

Which patients should be monitored?

Experts agree that continuous ST-segment monitoring is tremendously useful for detecting myocardial ischemia [1,2]. According to the Practice Standards for Electrocardiographic Monitoring in Hospital Settings, patients who are most likely to benefit from ST monitoring include those who are in the early phases of an acute coronary syndrome (ACS), those in the emergency department who are being monitored for chest pain or angina-type symptoms, those who have not achieved optimal reperfusion on angiogram following elective percutaneous coronary intervention (PCI), and those who suffer from variant angina. Therefore, these groups of patients are considered to have the highest priority for continuous ST-segment monitoring. ST monitoring also is recommended for the following groups of patients: patients with postacute MI, stable patients following elective PCI, patients who undergo surgery who are at risk for cardiac ischemia, and pediatric patients with a risk for MI or ischemia secondary to congenital or acquired conditions [2].

Patients who have suffered an acute coronary event, including MI or unstable angina, or who are being ruled in/out for MI are considered to have the greatest priority for ST-segment monitoring. Recom-

mended duration of monitoring is at least 24 hours, and until the patient has been event-free for 12 to 24 hours. Research shows that such monitoring may assist in (1) assessing coronary artery patency following reperfusion with thrombolytic therapy or PCI, (2) identifying acute closure after PCI, (3) recognizing recurrence of ischemia or infarct extension, and (4) noting transient ischemic events [2,11].

In the emergency department, patients who present with chest pain or other symptoms that could be indicative of an ACS may have no significant changes on the initial 12-lead ECG. With evolving MIs and dynamic changes in the ECG, the snapshot that a single 12-lead ECG provides may be nondiagnostic, even in true MI. Because this scenario could lead to a delay in the identification of ischemia and subsequent reperfusion, continuous ST monitoring is recommended for 8 to 12 hours in conjunction with serial cardiac biomarker testing to rule in or to rule out MI. Rule in patients may be treated more rapidly and rule out patients may avoid unnecessary hospital admissions.

Herren and colleagues [12] studied 383 patients who were admitted to the emergency room for chest pain. Patients were classified as low to moderate risk and had no additional signs or symptoms that were suggestive of MI. Continuous 12-lead ST-segment monitoring was implemented, combined with serial cardiac enzyme (creatine kinase MB) measurement. The researchers concluded that this methodology provided an accurate and effective way to rule out MI. Through this same method, two patients had the earliest possible diagnosis of acute evolving MI, and it facilitated the expeditious administration of thrombolytic medications.

Patients who have suboptimal angiographic results following PCI without an ACS should receive continuous ST-segment monitoring in the postprocedural period, because this is when they are most vulnerable to acute coronary reocclusion. Procedural complications, such as coronary artery dissection, intracoronary thrombosis, or simply less than desirable flow, may be contributing factors. If ST events occur during the monitoring period, the monitoring should continue for 24 hours or longer. Ideally, ST-segment monitoring is initiated in the cardiac catheterization laboratory, which allows identification of the ST fingerprint during balloon inflation [5]. This data could be reported to the nurse who is responsible for postprocedural care, who would monitor the patient in the best fingerprint lead; this would enhance the likelihood of detecting recurrent ischemia.

Individuals who present with possible variant angina may benefit from this technology because

ST-segments can be observed for transient elevation that is associated with coronary artery vasospasm. This may help to confirm the diagnosis, identify the anatomic location of the involved vessel, heighten awareness for dysrhythmia monitoring during anginal episodes, and determine the effectiveness of medical therapy. The suggested standard is to monitor patients who have variant angina for 12 to 24 hours after the initiation of therapy, barring any further ST events.

Although the recommendations are not as strong for the remaining groups of patients, ST- segment monitoring, if available, should be implemented. For patients who are in the postacute MI period, any new elevation in cardiac biomarkers, recurrence of chest pain, or other ischemic symptoms are reasons to continue ST-segment monitoring. If already discontinued, ST-segment monitoring should be resumed upon signs or symptoms of ischemia. ST-segment monitoring during activity can assist caregivers in determining the effectiveness of medication and the readiness for discharge [2].

Short-term ST-segment monitoring is recommended for 4 to 8 hours after uncomplicated, nonurgent PCI. Although significant postprocedural ST-segment findings are unlikely in this population, noncardiac symptoms, such as coronary "stretch" pain or gastrointestinal upset, can occur. The reassurance that ST-monitoring provides may help to exclude cardiac ischemia and to quell patient anxiety.

Following cardiac surgery, ST-segment monitoring could be helpful to differentiate types of pain (eg, incisional versus cardiac). Other suggested uses are to monitor graft patency and to assess for ischemia; however, evidence to support this is limited. In noncardiac surgical patients, individuals at risk for perioperative and postoperative ischemia could benefit from ST monitoring since etiology of myocardial ischemia may be coronary disease or increased myocardial oxygen demand; the latter can result from the effects of anesthesia or increased sympathetic stimulation during the postoperative waking period. For instance, researchers who explored the use of continuous intraoperative ST-segment monitoring during carotid endarterectomy concluded that the monitoring may be useful for the detection of myocardial ischemia. In a sample of 21 patients who underwent carotid endarterectomy, 1 patient had ST changes that resolved following the administration of nitroglycerin, and 2 other patients had ST-segment deviation that correlated to cross-clamping of the internal carotid artery [13].

Other research supported the usefulness of continuous intraoperative 12-lead ST-segment monitoring in patients who undergo major vascular surgery

[14]. In fact, even critically ill patients who do not undergo surgery and who have high myocardial oxygen demand may experience untoward cardiovascular events that could be detected by ST monitoring. This is particularly true in elderly patients [2]. Booker and colleagues [15] examined how often transient myocardial ischemia occurred in a sample of 76 noncardiac critically ill patients and found that 8 patients had a total of 37 ischemic events. Most of those events were silent, which reinforced the fact that chest pain is an unreliable indicator of ischemia. One finding supported that advanced age, transient myocardial ischemia, and elevated troponin values correlated significantly with cardiac complications.

One especially interesting area of research involves using ST-segment monitoring during weaning from mechanical ventilation as a method to predict weaning failure. ST segment changes that are suggestive of ischemia correlate with failure to wean [16,17]. This could be an immensely useful tool at the bedside to guide health care providers in determining patient tolerance of weaning trials.

Although there is little research to support ST-segment monitoring in the pediatric population, experts agree that certain groups of infants and children are at risk for ischemia and infarction [2]. Without abundant inquiry and technology to assist in fully understanding the use of ST-segment monitoring in pediatrics, this area warrants further exploration.

Which patients should not be monitored?

Despite the advantages of continuous ST-segment monitoring, it is not appropriate for all patients. Patient selection is crucial to avoid false alarms that can lead to nurse desensitization and fatigue [8]. Because patients with ECGs that show a left bundle-branch block pattern have distortion of the ST-segment, ST monitoring triggers false alarms. The ECG pattern of right bundle-branch block does not have the same degree of ST-segment distortion, which makes ST segment monitoring more practical [2,18]. Patients with ventricular pacemakers also have ST-segment changes that may trigger alarms inappropriately, even more so if the pacing is intermittent. Other rhythms that make ST-segment monitoring alarms less reliable—because of effects on the baseline ST—include intermittent idioventricular rhythm, coarse atrial flutter, or atrial fibrillation. Furthermore, pericarditis, electrolyte abnormalities, cardiac pre-excitation syndromes, and certain medications may skew the

ST segment. Despite this, some literature supports trending of ST-segment changes to monitor for silent myocardial ischemia, even in clinical situations that alter the appearance of the ST-segment [19]. Agitated or restless patients may show considerable artifact on the monitor. Likewise, confused patients who may remove the ECG electrodes or disconnect lead wires are difficult to monitor.

Measuring, analyzing, and interpreting the ST-segment

To use the data that are provided by ST-segment monitoring effectively, clinicians must know what to look for. This begins with an understanding of where to measure the ST-segment. ST-segment measurements are recorded as the number of millimeters of depression below, or elevation above, the isoelectric baseline. The reference for the isoelectric baseline is the T-P segment; it can be identified by putting a straight edge across the ECG from the end of the T wave to the beginning of the P wave. If the T-P segment cannot be distinguished easily, such as in tachyarrhythmias, the P-R segment may be used [20,21]. The J point is where the QRS complex ends, and returns to the patient's baseline ST segment. The ST segment should be measured 0.6 seconds after the J point. Although some sources suggested measuring at 0.8 seconds after the J point, the 0.6-second mark is less likely to be skewed by the initial deflection of the T-wave. ST elevation or depression of 1 to 2 mm that lasts for at least 1 minute can be clinically significant and warrants further patient assessment [1,3,8]. The key to monitoring ST-segments lies in trending deviation from each patient's baseline ST-segment and determining whether this may be clini-cally significant. Fig. 1 shows a normal ST segment with reference points and examples of ST depression and elevation.

Which leads should be monitored?

Ideally, a monitoring system is able to monitor ST-segments of all 12 leads at once. A 12-lead display, printing capability, and a full-disclosure system that allows retrospective review also are desirable features. Three lead configurations are available that can provide derived or modified 12-lead ECG data [2]. These configurations vary from the traditional static 12-lead ECG so a side-by-side comparison is not appropriate [22]. For patients who have inferior wall MI who sustained concomitant right ventricular MI, right-sided chest leads may be used [19].

Although monitoring all leads provides the most valuable and comprehensive information, many organizations are limited to monitoring systems with five electrodes, which permits a maximum of seven leads to be displayed at once, only one of which is a precordial (V) lead. Some monitoring equipment now has the capability to monitor a second V lead by way of a sixth lead wire. Recommendations for which leads to monitor are summarized in Table 1 [1–3,8,19,22]. Ideally, the anatomic site of ischemia or the lead that is indicative of the individual's ST fingerprint should determine the leads that are selected for display. If neither is known, leads III and V_3 should be used for monitoring patients who experience an ACS. If a second precordial lead can be monitored, the addition of V_5 is recommended [3,22].

When 12-lead monitoring is unavailable, the ST fingerprint has not been identified, but the culprit vessel for supplying the ischemic myocardium is

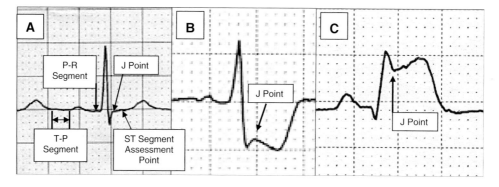

Fig. 1. (*A*) A normal ECG complex shows T-P segment and P-R segment, which may be used as reference points to the isoelectric line. The ST-segment is measured at 0.6 seconds after the J point. This ST-segment is isoelectric. (*B*) ECG complex show ST-segment depression of almost 5 mm. (*C*) ST-segment elevation of approximately 4 mm is depicted.

Table 1
Which leads to monitor as related to anatomy

	Anterior MI	Inferior MI	Lateral MI	Posterior MI
Usual vessel	Left anterior descending artery	Right coronary artery	Circumflex or right coronary artery	Right coronary artery
Leads to monitor	V2	III	No definitive lead	Reciprocal leads: V1, V2, V3
	V3	aVF		
	V4	II	Consider V5, V6	

known, lead selection should be specific to the involved coronary artery. For monitoring the right coronary artery (inferior wall) the best lead to monitor is lead III, followed by lead aVF, and thirdly, lead II. Despite expert recommendations that are based on clinical studies that showed that lead II is not the best lead to observe unless it is the patient's ST fingerprint, it remains the most commonly monitored lead in critical care units across the nation [4]. When monitoring the left anterior descending (LAD) artery (anterior wall), lead V2 or V3 is best. V4 also may reflect anterior wall ischemia, but is not as sensitive. For occlusions that involve the left circumflex artery, ST-segment changes may be seen in the inferior, lateral, or posterior leads. Therefore, no lead is definitive for a circumflex occlusion, although some literature supports using leads V5 and V6 to detect lateral wall ischemia or leads II, III, and aVF to observe for circumflex-dependent inferior wall ischemia. Posterior wall ischemia may be detected by looking for the reciprocal changes of ST-segment depression in leads V1, V2, and V3 [1,8,22].

Strategies for clinical success

Interdisciplinary collaboration

Monitoring of the ECG is primarily a nursing function; however, some organizations rely on physicians to direct which parameters are monitored and considered significant. Because of this, it is critical that interdisciplinary collaboration occurs when reviewing evidence and making decisions about ECG monitoring so that everyone can support best practice.

Evaluating monitoring equipment

To monitor ST-segment changes effectively, cardiac-monitoring equipment should have ST-segment analysis software and ST-segment alarm capabilities. If purchasing new equipment, consideration of a moni-

toring system with continuous 12-lead capabilities would add value for ST-monitoring. ST-segment alarms should not require manual configuration by the bedside caregiver. Instead, alarms should be set to go off with 1- or 2-mm deviations from the patient's baseline, unless—based on the individual patient's needs and the professional nurse's judgment—the alarms need to be modified or disabled.

Other factors to explore when purchasing monitoring equipment include evaluating how much technical, educational, and training support the vendor will provide. Discussion of the ability for future equipment upgrades and the vendor's commitment to customer service should occur.

The group that evaluates new monitors should be multidisciplinary, and should include physicians, nurses, information technology personnel, and biomedical engineers. If the care model includes the use of monitoring technicians, consideration should be given to which equipment will support such practice most effectively. A crucial factor to include in planning is how monitor technicians will communicate with the nurses, particularly if the monitor technicians are housed in a location that is remote or separate from the patient care area. Possibilities include telephones, pagers, nurse locator systems, and wireless messaging devices.

Physician participation may help to maximize future medical staff support. Physician involvement in decisions about cardiac monitoring vary from facility to facility. If monitoring changes are planned in a variety of clinical areas, then the appropriate medical staff should be involved in those discussions. For example, if changes are to be made in the operating room, it is be crucial to include anesthesiologists in the decision-making process.

Involved nursing personnel should include administrators or managers with budgetary responsibility, advanced practice nurses, and front-line caregivers. Encouraging staff nurses, who will be applying the technology directly, to participate in the evaluation of equipment can be crucial to identifying ease of use, process issues, and clinical practicality. Staff nurses

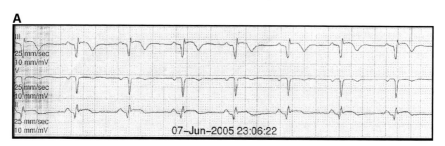

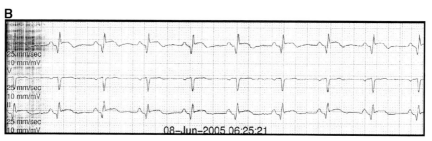

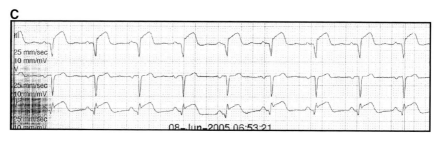

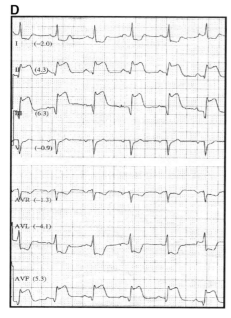

also can be effective champions in facilitating practice changes on a peer-to-peer basis, and will feel valued for having been consulted.

Biomedical engineers are important team members because they possess great knowledge about equipment and typically are responsible for maintenance and repair. Likewise, information technology staff can assist in determining whether new monitoring equipment can interface with other information systems that are in use and can help to plan for the future. With automated documentation systems fully implemented in many facilities and in the planning stages for more yet, the ability of bedside monitors to communicate with and download information to other systems is essential.

Another consideration is whether the system can be used seamlessly across the care continuum. This type of process allows data to travel with the patient through different levels of care, such as when transferring from the ICU to telemetry. This approach helps to avoid fragmented information and promotes continuity of care. One key point is that the evaluation should not focus solely on how cardiac monitoring is done today, but what it might look like over the next decade or longer.

False alarms

Clinical staff often cites false alarms as major irritants. Chronic overstimulation can lead to staff fatigue; desensitization to alarms may result. A possible consequence is missed alarms, which could lead to unfavorable patient outcomes.

Several practices can help to minimize false alarms: correct skin preparation; consistent lead placement, individualizing alarms to each patient, and awareness of the effect of body position on ST-recordings [2,3]. Skin preparation is important to reduce skin resistance and can be minimized by abrading the skin

mildly. Several commercially available products can be used or it can be accomplished by wiping the skin surface with gauze, a washcloth, or a paper towel. Shaving off hair at electrode sites and cleansing with alcohol or soap and water can assist by removing oil and dead skin cells. Care should be taken not to use excess alcohol because it can have a drying effect on the skin, which reduces conduction. Before application, the gel patch in the center of each electrode should be checked to ensure that it is moist [2,3,8,23]. Leaving electrodes out of original packaging and exposed to air can promote premature dehydration of the conductive gel.

Consistent and accurate lead placement helps to provide consistent ECG information; therefore, electrode sites should be marked with indelible ink so that if electrodes are removed, new ones can be placed in the same location. Changing the location of precordial leads as little as 1 cm can alter the ECG waveform [1–3]. It is important that all staff who may be responsible for applying electrodes be informed of the importance of accurate lead placement and receive training to support consistent practice.

Individualizing alarms to the patient can help to minimize inappropriate alarms. The monitor should be set to alarm when ST changes of 1 to 2 mm from the patient's baseline occur, rather than deviation from the isoelectric line [8]. The clinician also must be able to distinguish whether the ST-segment change is clinically significant for new ischemia or whether it represents a normalizing of the ST-segment because of reperfusion. Some patients have ST-segments that are not isoelectric because of nonischemic-related causes, such as digitalis, which can produce ST-segment depression [21]. In contrast, pericarditis may produce widespread ST-segment elevation on the ECG.

Position of the patient when doing the ST-segment reading is important. Recommended practice is to measure the ST while the patient is supine and the

---

Fig. 2. Case study. M.A. was transferred from a community hospital a few hours following thrombolytic treatment for an acute inferior MI. His history was significant for acute inferior MI 1 week before this readmission for which he had a stent placed in his right coronary artery (RCA), as well as a known 100% occlusion of his middle left anterior descending artery. He was taken urgently to the cardiac catheterization lab where 100% reocclusion of his RCA was discovered, and two drug-eluting stents were placed with successful reperfusion. (*A*) ECG waveforms several hours after his procedure show ST-segment elevation of approximately 1 mm in leads III and II with T-wave inversion. (*B*) The following morning at 0625 his ST segments largely were unchanged. (*C*) At approximately 0650, the ST segment alarms on the telemetry monitoring system began sounding. ST-segment elevation of almost 4 mm is visible in lead III along with ST elevation of 3 mm in lead II. The nurse checked the patient, who had no symptoms; notified the physician; and administered nitroglycerin sublingually. Approximately 10 minutes later, the patient developed severe chest pain and shortness of breath. (*D*) Full view of all leads available at that time with ST elevation of over 6 mm in lead III, 5 mm in aVF, and 4 mm in lead II. Reciprocal ST-segment depression can be seen in leads I and aVL. M.A. was transferred emergently to the cardiac catheterization lab where the proximal RCA was found to be 100% occluded with clots throughout. An intraaortic balloon pump was placed, and he went to the operating room for coronary artery bypass grafting. M.A. was discharged from the hospital on his seventh postoperative day after an uncomplicated recovery.

head of the bed is elevated to a maximum of 45°. When a ST-segment alarm sounds, the nurse should check the patient's position and return him to the supine position if the patient has moved. ST alarms that persist upon return to the supine position should be regarded as related to ischemia [3].

Knowledge and training

In basic ECG training, emphasis typically is placed on monitoring for cardiac dysrhythmias, and less time is spent on the ST-segment changes that are associated with acute coronary syndromes. Monitor technicians and nurses may be involved in ECG monitoring. Several key issues need to be addressed in training those who are responsible for watching monitors, interpreting ECGs, and assessing and intervening upon patients. These include how to measure and interpret ST-segments, the significance of ST-segment changes, how to use monitoring equipment correctly, alarm management, electrode positioning, application and maintenance, and actions to take when ST-alarms occur. The implications that ST-segment monitoring has in relation to patient outcomes should be clear to everyone. One strategy that has been effective in staff education is the presentation of case studies that demonstrate how ST-segment monitoring affects patients who have been cared for in their own clinical practice setting [21]. Understanding the impact that nursing expertise in ECG and ST-segment monitoring can have on patient outcomes is imperative. Case studies that highlight nursing interventions, in particular—that allowed for early recognition and treatment of myocardial ischemia—can be powerful. Fig. 2 shows a case example of acute closure that was detected with ST-segment monitoring.

ECG monitoring may be done in a variety of settings across the continuum, including the emergency department; procedural areas, such as the cardiac catheterization laboratory; operating rooms; critical care units; progressive care areas; telemetry units; or medical-surgical divisions. This monitoring involves a variety of staff with a corresponding variety of expertise, and may extend beyond nurses to monitor technicians. It is important to consider all areas in the hospital where cardiac monitoring is done to ensure that appropriate staff training occurs and to promote seamless ECG monitoring.

Minimum competency for staff that participates in ECG monitoring should be defined, and then theoretic and practical training should be designed to help achieve the expected competency. After training

and practice, assessment should occur to validate that learning occurred and clinical guidelines are being followed. Reassessing competency periodically to validate knowledge retention and application is essential to quality care.

Summary

To implement a change in practice, the involved clinicians must appreciate the value and practicality of any type of monitoring. There is significant research in the nursing and medical literature to support the use of continuous ST-segment monitoring in a variety of clinical settings and situations; this lays the foundation for true patient care–driven decision making. Nurse and physician experts have issued guidelines for ST-segment ECG monitoring. As patient advocates, nurses are compelled to act in the best interests of their patients. Now is the time to evaluate whether ST-segment monitoring is done as the guidelines suggest. If yes, nurses can be confident that the best available care is being offered to patients. If not, the bar has been raised and nurses must rise to the challenge.

References

[1] Drew BJ, Krucoff MW. Multilead ST-segment monitoring in patients with acute coronary syndromes; a consensus statement for healthcare professionals. ST-Segment Monitoring Practice Guideline International Working Group. Am J Crit Care 1999; 8(6):372–88.
[2] Drew BJ, Califf RM, Funk M, et al. Practice standards for electrocardiographic monitoring in hospital settings. Circulation 2004;110(17):2721–46.
[3] American Association of Critical Care Nurses. Practice alert: ST segment monitoring. Available at: http://www.aacn.org//AACN/practiceAlert.nsf/Files/ECG%20ST%20Segment/$file/ECG%20ST%20Segment.pdf. Accessed March 11, 2005.
[4] Patton JA, Funk M. Survey of use of ST-segment monitoring in patients with acute coronary syndromes. Am J Crit Care 2001;10(1):23–34.
[5] Krucoff MW, Parente AR, Bottner RK, et al. Stability of multilead ST-segment "fingerprints" over time after percutaneous transluminal coronary angioplasty and its usefulness in detecting reocclusion. Am J Cardiol 1988;61:1232–7.
[6] Caldwell MA, Pelter MM, Drew BJ. Chest pain is an unreliable measure of ischemia in men and women during PTCA. Heart Lung 1996;25(6):423–9.
[7] Fesmire FM, Percy RF, Bardoner JB, et al. Usefulness of automated serial 12-lead ECG monitoring dur-

ing the initial emergency department evaluation of patients with chest pain. Ann Emerg Med 1998;31(1): 3–11.

[8] Leeper B. Continuous ST-segment monitoring. AACN Clin Issues Crit Care Nurs 2003;14(2):145–54.

[9] Pelter MM, Adams MG, Drew BJ. Transient myocardial ischemia is an independent predictor of adverse in-hospital outcomes in patients with acute coronary syndromes treated in the telemetry unit. Heart Lung 2003;32(2):71–8.

[10] Patel DJ, Holdwright DR, Knight CJ, et al. Early continuous ST segment monitoring in unstable angina: prognostic value additional to the clinical characteristics and the admission electrocardiogram. Heart 1996;75(3):222–8.

[11] Klootwijk P, Cobbaert C, Fioretti P, et al. Noninvasive assessment of reperfusion and reocclusion after thrombolysis in acute myocardial infarction. Am J Cardiol 1993;72:75G–84G.

[12] Herren KR, Mackway-Jones K, Richards CR, et al. Is it possible to exclude a diagnosis of myocardial damage within six hours of admission to an emergency department? Diagnostic cohort study. BMJ 2001;323(7309):372–4.

[13] Kawahito S, Kitahata H, Tanaka K, et al. Dynamic QRS-complex and ST-segment monitoring by continuous vectorcardiography during carotid endarterectomy. Br J Anaesth 2003;90(2):142–7.

[14] Landesberg G, Mosseri M, Wolf Y, et al. Perioperative myocardial ischemia and infarction: identification by continuous 12-lead electrocardiogram with on-line ST-segment monitoring. Anesthesiology 2002;96(2): 264–70.

[15] Booker KJ, Holm K, Drew BJ, et al. Frequency and outcomes of transient myocardial ischemia in critically ill adults admitted for noncardiac conditions. Am J Crit Care 2003;12(6):508–17.

[16] Chatila W, Ani S, Guanglione D, et al. Cardiac ischemia during weaning from mechanical ventilation. Chest 1996;109(6):1577–83.

[17] Srivastava S, Chatila W, Amoateng-Adjepong Y, et al. Myocardial ischemia and weaning failure in patients with coronary artery disease: an update. Crit Care Med 1999;27(10):2109–12.

[18] Pelter MM, Adams MG. ST segment changes in right bundle branch block. Am J Crit Care 2005;14(4): 341–2.

[19] Bell NN. Clinical significance of ST-segment monitoring. Crit Care Nurs Clin North Am 1992;4(2):313–23.

[20] Conover MB. Normal electrical activation of the heart. In: Conover MB, editor. Understanding electrocardiography. 8th edition. St. Louis (MO): Mosby; 2003. p. 8–22.

[21] Graf C, Drew BJ. Continuous ST segment monitoring: how it works. Am J Nurse 1993;93(Suppl):18S–22S.

[22] Delaiden AM, Schell H. Setting a new gold standard. ST-segment monitoring provides early detection of myocardial ischemia. Am J Nurse 2003;101(Suppl): 4S–8S.

[23] Clochesy JM, Cifani L, Howe K. Electrode site preparation techniques: a follow up study. Heart Lung 1991; 20(1):27–30.

ELSEVIER
SAUNDERS

Crit Care Nurs Clin N Am 18 (2006) 179–187

CRITICAL CARE
NURSING CLINICS
OF NORTH AMERICA

Arterial Pressure–Based Technologies: A New Trend in Cardiac Output Monitoring

Jan M. Headley, RN, BS

Edwards Lifesciences LLC, One Edwards Way, Irvine, CA 91264, USA

The use of arterial pressure as an indirect method of determining cardiac output (CO) is not new; however, with recent improvements in signal extraction, microprocessing, and sophisticated algorithms, the technology is gaining more clinical acceptance [1–4]. When adopting a new technology into practice, three key questions need to be answered: (1) is the method technologically sound?, (2) is it based on physiological principles?, and (3) are the applications clinically important? As with any technology that is used in the care of patients, the indications, applications, and potential limitations also must be understood.

Blood pressure monitoring provides only part of the hemodynamic assessment that is needed to manage the critically ill. Organ (tissue) perfusion is determined not so much by pressure, but more so by flow, or CO [4,5]. Technologies that are based on the arterial pressure provide CO determinations and other clinically important variables, such as stroke volume variation (SVV), pulse pressure variation (PPV), and systolic pressure variation (SPV). Clinical use of these parameters is emerging as a means for determining the patient's ability to respond to fluid [6–9].

Is the method technologically sound?

Theory behind arterial pulse technologies

The underlying theory that is applied to arterial pulse technologies is founded on the concept that

stroke volume (SV) may be derived from the arterial pressure or the pulse waveform. This theory is refined by two principles: (1) aortic pulse pressure (PP)—the difference between systolic pressure (SP) and diastolic pressure (DP)—is proportional to SV, and (2) PP is inversely proportional to aortic compliance [10–13]. After SV is determined, the arterial pulsations are counted to determine the heart rate (HR). CO is expressed as HR multiplied by SV (CO = HR × SV) [10,11,14].

Threats to the proportionality of SV to PP assumption are related directly to vessel compliance and peripheral vascular changes. Aortic compliance and peripheral resistance are affected by factors that change vessel stiffness, or cause vasoconstriction or vasodilation. These effects can occur rapidly, and subsequently, impact the arterial waveform, and potentially, arterial pressures [15]. The interactions between SP, PP, compliance, and resistance—otherwise known as vessel or vasomotor tone—are complex and cannot be described by a single mechanism [13,16]. A further explanation of these interactions is described later.

Currently available arterial-based technologies

Various methods exist—which incorporate some form of waveform, pressure assessment, or both in the algorithms—for determining CO from the arterial pulse [1–4,17]. Until recently, two commercially available methods were described as pulse contour (based on arterial waveform) and pulse power (based on the mean arterial pressure; MAP). Concerns and limitations revolve around the obtainment of accurate arterial waveforms or the requirement for additional calibration [1,2,4,17,18].

E-mail address: jan.headley@edwards.com

Methods that are based on more simple models of the arterial system assume consistent pressures throughout the vascular tree, nonchanging aortic properties, and steady vascular resistance. The overall values were less than precise [18,19]. To accommodate for physiologic changes, external calibration methods are required. Available technologies that require calibration include the LiDCO system (LiDCO Group [20]), which uses lithium as the calibration medium for indicator dilution techniques, and the PiCCO system (Pulsion SG [21]), which uses a transpulmonary thermodilution technique that requires central vessel access, a femoral line, and a large bolus of cooled solution as the thermal indicator. Because additional invasive lines are required for calibration, the usefulness of these systems is limited [1,2,4,18].

A newly available technology for arterial pressure CO (APCO) determination also is based on the assessment of arterial pulse waveform and PPs. A robust algorithm compensates for the individual patient's vessel compliance and changes in vascular tone, and thereby, does not require additional external calibration [17]. The system uses the patient's existing arterial catheter, which is attached to a sensor. This sensor (FloTrac, Edwards Lifesciences LLC, Irvine, California [22]) has a bifurcated cable with one going to the bedside monitor to display arterial pressures and the other going to the Vigileo (Edwards Lifesciences LLC [22]) monitor to collect and analyze the arterial pressures for CO determinations. Fig. 1 shows the FloTrac and Vigileo system.

With FloTrac, arterial pressures are measured at a sampling rate of 100 Hz (times per second) over a 20-second period, which provides approximately 2000 data points. The variations of the pressure are analyzed mathematically to determine the SD. The SD of the PP is proportional more precisely to SV, in that multiple values are measured to determine the variability, rather than a simple single SP and DP for the PP component. Factors that affect larger vessel compliance, such as age, gender, height, and weight, are input into the Vigileo monitor. Changes in the patient's vascular tone are compensated for by internal waveform analysis [14,17]. Partly because of the robust algorithm, specific patient changes are evaluated, and therefore, external calibration is not required [17,23–25].

This new less invasive technology satisfies three key physiologic requirements of assessing CO with an arterial pulse: PP is proportional to SV, aortic compliance changes are compensated for, and alterations in vascular tone are assessed. Comparison studies with various patient populations and conditions and with wide CO values showed the FloTrac system to be comparable to intermittent thermodilution bolus and continuous CO technologies [23–25].

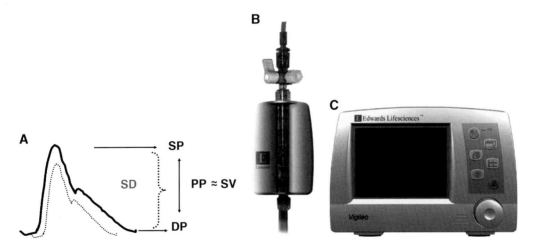

Fig. 1. (*A*) The solid line represents the arterial waveform. The difference between the SP and DP is PP, which is proportional to SV. By counting the amplitudes, the HR is determined. HR × SV = CO. The dotted line reflects the arterial pulse measured at 100 Hz. Variability of the arterial pressure waveform is made over a 20 second period. This variability is the SD of all the pressure. SD is more precise in determining the proportionality of PP to SV. (*B*) The FloTrac sensor on the left is attached to the patient's existing arterial line. A bifurcated cable attaches the sensor to the bedside monitor pressure connector and the other to the Vigileo monitor where the CO value is displayed on a continuous basis (*C*). (Fig. 1B and 1C, Courtesy of Edwards Lifesciences LLC, Irvine, CA; with permission.)

Is the technology based on physiologic principles?

Pressure, resistance, and flow interrelationships

In the clinical arena, CO typically is described as HR times SV. The interrelationships of pressure (P), resistance (R), and flow (F) become the descriptors when using arterial-based technologies for CO determinations. Clinically, the assessment variables for P, R, and F are systemic blood pressure, calculated systemic vascular resistance, and CO [5,10,11]. Fig. 2 illustrates how the common equation of CO = HR × SV can be rearranged to evaluate the interrelationship of P, R, and F. This relationship provides an understanding of how CO also is determined by the interaction between P and R. Another descriptor of vessel resistance is vascular tone, which includes compliance and resistance [5,26]. Therefore, CO can be evaluated by the following equation: CO = P/R [5,11].

Physiologic factors that affect the arterial pulse

Three key mechanisms affect the arterial blood pressure. They are divided into those that impact the pulse wave itself, the pressures that are produced from the wave, and the waveform that is generated and displayed. Arterial blood pressure is determined by SV and vascular tone. When the left ventricular (LV) SV increases or the vascular tone increases, the typical result is an increase in SP. A decrease in SP results if the LV SV decreases or if vascular tone becomes more compliant. The interactions of LV SV, compliance characteristics of the vascular system, and vessel tone are complex [1,26,27].

Pressures that are produced from the arterial pulse wave contain four values: SP, DP, PP, and mean. Two components make up the arterial pulse: the pulsatile component consists of the PP, and MAP is the steady component. A phenomenon of wave amplification occurs in the vascular tree, which produces an elevated SP as the wave travels into more distal branches. As the waves become amplified and produce a higher presser, the actual blood flow diminishes; however, the mean value is not affected greatly [13,27]. Because the newest APCO device is not dependent on the SP pressure and incorporates the SD of the full arterial waveform, various arterial line insertion sites may be used that will provide continuous CO values [24].

The arterial waveform consists of three components: (1) the forward flow wave, also called incident wave; (2) the dicrotic notch, which reflects aortic valve closure; and (3) the reflective, backward, wave. Alterations in the morphology of the waveform occur, in part, as a result of factors that affect the pulse components [27,28]. The aorta modulates the amplitude of the pressure that results from ventricular ejection. The amount of modulation depends on the compliance of the aorta. The less compliant the aorta, the less modulation; therefore, a higher pressure is generated. The more compliant the aorta, the more modulation occurs, which produces a lesser pressure. The net result is to dampen the pulsatile flow from the left ventricle. This modulation effect is called the "Windkessel effect" and impacts the arterial waveform and subsequent pressure [27–29].

In conditions such as aging, arterial hypertension, arteriosclerosis, diabetes, and heart failure, aortic compliance decreases, which produces an increase in SPs and PP [27]. Therefore, factors that affect aortic compliance need to be considered with the APCO technology; subsequently, the patient's age, gender, height, and weight are input into the Vigileo to make the results more precise for the individual patient [14,17].

The second component of the arterial wave, the dicrotic notch, is used often as a demarcation of the closure of the aortic valve to identify the end of systole and the onset of diastole [10]. The dicrotic notch does not always coincide with actual aortic valve closure. Stiffening of the peripheral vessel that occurs with age, disease processes, and with certain therapeutic agents impacts the backward reflective wave. As a result, the dicrotic notch may occur higher up on the descent of the arterial pressure wave, which makes it more difficult to determine exact closure of the aortic valve [27,28]. Techniques for SV assessment that rely on dicrotic notch identification (eg, pulse contour) may be impacted by reflective waves. This physiologic fact requires additional calculations with the use of pulse contour to determine where the dicrotic notch occurs [1,2,30]. Fig. 3 shows the impact of a large reflective wave on the location of

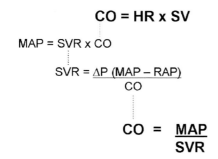

Fig. 2. Pressure, resistance, and flow interrelationships.

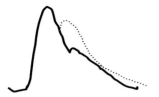

Fig. 3. Impact of reflective wave on location of dicrotic notch. Impact of reflective waves on arterial pulse waveform. Solid line represents a normal arterial waveform. Dotted line reflects the potential impact of a reflective wave on the dicrotic notch. The reflective wave alters the identification of the location of the dicrotic notch.

the dicrotic notch; it makes it difficult to identify aortic valve closure.

The theory behind arterial–pressure based technology is based on the premise of PP being proportional to SV. Threats to the proportionality of SV and PP include the effects of altered aortic compliance and changing vascular resistance. Aortic compliance is inversely proportional to PP [5,6,12,13]. Decreased compliance stiffens the vessels, which increases SP. An increased SP with no change in DP widens the PP. SP may increase as a result of increased vessel stiffness; however, the increase in PP may not be caused by an increase in SV. SP depends not only on LV SV but also on vessel compliance and

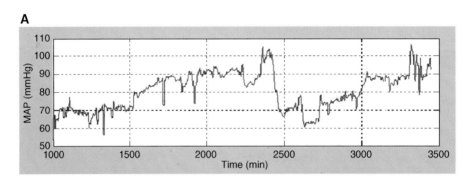

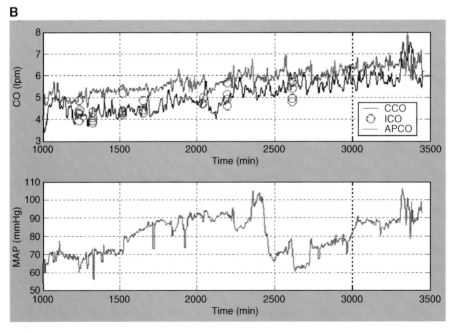

Fig. 4. Trend over time of MAP and APCO. Does MAP equal CO? If only the MAP is assessed (*trend A*), the increase in MAP might lead the clinician to trust that the CO had increased as well, and that when the MAP dropped precipitously, the CO would have dropped as well. When observing both trends (*trend B*), the CO increased with the decrease in MAP. Light line, APCO; dark line, continuous CO (CCO) by thermodilution; open circle, intermittent thermodilution CO boluses.

DP (SP = PP + DP). Therefore, SP is related less closely to SV than is PP [6,13].

Changes in vascular tone affect the arterial waveform and may impact SPs and DPs. The effect of vascular resistance changes on the arterial waveform need to be accommodated for so as not to violate APCO principles [1,2]. PP for any given ventricular ejection and HR depend on arterial compliance, and the timing and magnitude of peripheral pulse wave reflection [30].

Are the applications clinically important?

Pressure does not always equal flow

Determining CO is an important component of care in the patients who have compromised cardio-vascular function [31,32]. Blood pressure does not reflect blood flow directly, but rather has an inter-connected relationship (P = F × R); therefore, all components necessitate assessment [4,5]. Fig. 4 demonstrates a patient in whom MAP and CO were being monitored continuously. Over a period of time the MAP exhibited a slow increase and then a precipitous decrease. With an assumption of pressure and flow being linear, the conclusion is that as MAP increases so does the CO, and when MAP decreases so does the CO. In this study, note that when MAP increased there was an increase in CO as measured by the APCO system; however, when the precipitous decrease occurred, the CO continued to increase. Without the additional CO information, there may have been an unnecessary intervention to increase CO.

Arterial pressure–based parameters assess fluid responsiveness

Additional clinically important variables that are obtained by arterial pressure–based techniques are indices that help to determine the patient's ability to respond to fluid resuscitation [4,6–9]. Volume resuscitation is an important maneuver in caring for critically ill patients. Traditional pressure-based parameters to assess the patient's preload status may be misleading. Volumetric parameters, such as end-diastolic volume, are more accurate indicators of preload than is pressure [33,34]. Being able to assess preload accurately does not necessarily predict the patient's ability to respond to increased preload or fluid administration [6,30,31].

Pulmonary artery catheter–obtained and -derived parameters are used to evaluate the response to fluid with varying results. Studies have found that pressure-based indices, such as central venous pressure, right atrial pressures, and pulmonary artery occlusion pressures, are not good predictors of response to fluid [33–35]. Newer arterial pressure–based parameters that are being studied to achieve this include SVV and its surrogates, SPV and PPV. Box 1 lists the parameters, descriptions, and equations. These indices assess the patient's response to fluid administration, and more importantly, predict if they will be responsive to fluid. Often, giving fluid to a patient who would not benefit from it is costly, not only to the patient in the form of potential fluid overload, increased morbidity, or mortality, but to the hospital as an unnecessary expense [7–9,30,32].

Physiology that supports parameters that assess fluid responsiveness

Pulsus paradoxus, defined as a greater than 5 to 10 mm Hg decrease in SP at the end of inspiration to the SP value at the end of expiration, is the basis of determining fluid responsiveness. This phenomenon may be associated with conditions such as asthma, hypovolemia, cardiac tamponade, and others. By continuously monitoring invasive arterial pressure, the increase and decrease of SP during the respiratory cycle is observed more easily in the critically ill patient. The excessive undulations in the arterial

---

Box 1. Arterial pressure – based parameters for assessing fluid responsiveness

Systolic pressure variation (mm Hg): difference between the maximum and minimum values of systolic arterial pressure recorded over a single respiratory cycle. Normal value is less than 10 mm Hg.
SPMax – SPMin
Pulse pressure variation (%): measured over a single respiratory cycle and defined as the maximal PP (SP – DP) less the minimal PP divided by the mean of these two pressures. Normal value is less than 13%.
(PPMax – PPMin)/PPmean
Stroke Volume Variation (%): measured over a single respiratory cycle and defined as the maximal stroke volume less the minimal stroke volume divided by the mean of these two stroke volumes. Normal value is less than 10%.
(SVMax – SVMin)/SVmean

waveform have been used as a clinical sign of the patient's need for fluid [6,8,9,36,37].

Heart–lung interactions are complex and subtle under different physiologic and mechanical respiratory conditions. It is beyond the scope of this article to review the intricacies of the interactions, which are described well in other papers [6–9,32,34]. A brief description follows to provide a basic understanding of the impact of respiration on the heart–lung mechanics.

Under normal conditions, and with spontaneous breathing, arterial blood pressure fluctuates throughout the respiratory cycle; it decreases with inspiration and increases with expiration. Intrathoracic pressure (ITP) changes that occur during respiration are transmitted to the heart chambers, pulmonary vascular bed, and great vessels. During inspiration, there is a decrease in ITP that causes an increase in venous return. The right ventricle (RV) dilates to accom-

modate this increase in preload. This results in an increase in RV stroke output into the compliant pulmonary vascular bed, where, as a result of decreased pressure, blood is sequestered. This decreases the amount of blood volume to the left side of the heart for filling with a subsequent decrease in LV SV. The end product is a decrease in SP. During expiration the converse occurs. A higher ITP is generated, which decreases venous return, RV filling, and RV SV. The sequestered blood in the pulmonary vasculature is diverted into the left side of the heart during the expiratory phase, which produces a higher LV SV and increased SP [6–9,35,37,38]. This interaction occurs over a full respiratory cycle that consists of a few seconds and a few heartbeats; during this period, the RV and left ventricle eject different blood volumes. The differing amounts equilibrate over a short period of time; this is not significant for patients who have normal physiology [32,37].

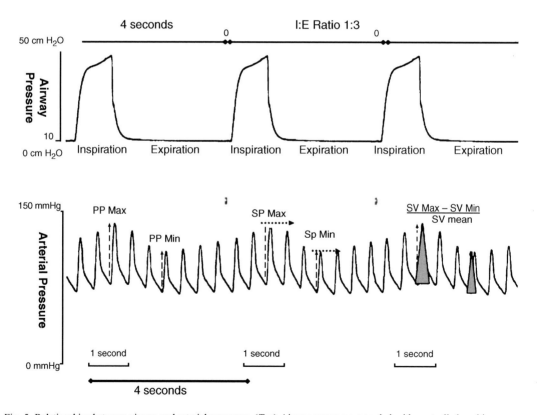

Fig. 5. Relationships between airway and arterial pressures. (*Top*) Airway pressures recorded with controlled positive pressure mechanical ventilation. Inspiration (I) is recorded as a positive wave. During expiration (E) the pressures return to baseline; however, they do not go below that or become negative. (*Bottom*) All of the parameters are measured at the peak point during inspiration and at the lowest point during expiration. The values are compared over the full respiratory cycle to determine the difference. PP Max, PP (SP − DP) at peak point during inspiration; PP Min, PP (SP − DP) at lowest point during expiration; SP Max, SP at peak point during inspiration; SP Min, SP at lowest point during expiration; SV Max, filled triangle denotes SV at peak point during inspiration; SV Min, filled triangle denotes SV at lowest point during expiration.

The sequela of heart–lung interactions is reversed from normal with controlled mechanical ventilation. During a controlled mechanical breath, the pressures increase with inspiration and decline during expiration. Increased ITP causes decreased RV venous return and increased RV afterload, which effectively decrease LV filling after a lag of two to three heart beats to allow for pulmonary vascular transit time [38]. With hypovolemic states, the variation between inspiration and expiration becomes greater than normal. This phenomenon often has been termed "reverse pulsus paradoxus" or respirator paradox [6]. Therefore, the use of SPV, PPV, or SVV for preload responsiveness determination are best performed under mechanical ventilation because the amount of tidal volume, respiratory rate, and positive pressure influences are controlled [38,39]. Fig. 5 depicts the relationships between airway pressure and arterial pressures during the respiratory cycle and the various parameters for assessment of fluid responsiveness.

Indications for the use of SPV, PPV, or SVV are evaluation of the patient's response to fluid administration and determination or prediction of the patient's ability to respond to fluids. Fig. 6 illustrates a case in which the SVV values were used to determine the patient's need for fluid and response to volume administration. Recall that SV is propor-

tional to PP. SVV is the primary parameter that indicates the ability to respond to fluid, and PPV and SPV are the pressure-based surrogates. Research showed that SPV, PPV, and SVV have reasonable correlations [6,8,13,37–39]. Typically, the greater the variability, the more likely it is that the patient requires fluid and will be responsive to it. Identified target values are SPV of greater than 10 mm Hg, PPV of greater than 13%, and SVV of greater than 10% [39]. Other researchers reported overall ranges for fluid responsiveness to be 10% to 15% [37]. Limitations are related directly to conditions that affect ITP, subsequent venous return, and cardiac filling. Patients who are breathing spontaneously and who have varying tidal volumes are not candidates for reproducible SVV values at this time because ITP is altered during breathing. The effects of other factors that need to be researched are changes in respiratory rate, tidal volume, positive end-expiratory pressure, and irregular heart rhythms [4,32–34].

Technical factors that affect the arterial waveform

Because these newer CO assessment methods are based on arterial pressure, factors that influence the quality of the pressure waveforms may produce

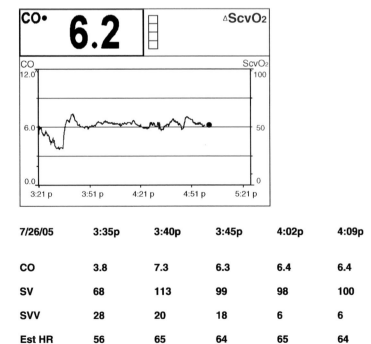

7/26/05	3:35p	3:40p	3:45p	4:02p	4:09p
CO	3.8	7.3	6.3	6.4	6.4
SV	68	113	99	98	100
SVV	28	20	18	6	6
Est HR	56	65	64	65	64

Fig. 6. A case in which the SVV values were used to determine the patient's need for fluid and response to volume administration.

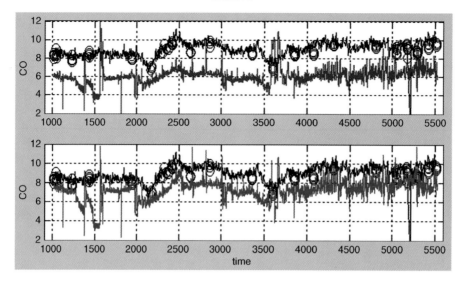

Fig. 7. A case in which the level of the FloTrac sensor was incorrect and the impact that it had on subsequent APCO determinations. In the top portion, the dark line represents the comparative thermodilution CO trend and the lighter line, APCO. The APCO sensor was found to be misaligned from the phlebostatic axis. In the bottom portion of the trend graph, the values were corrected for proper sensor alignment. Notice how the two values became closer once arterial pressures were being measured accurately.

erroneous values. Proper pressure system set-up, leveling of the sensor, and zeroing techniques assist with ensuring optimal pressure recordings [1]. Fig. 7 shows a case in which the level of the FloTrac sensor was incorrect and the impact that it had on subsequent APCO determinations. With the misalignment, the pressures that were obtained by the sensor did not reflect the patient's arterial pressures and led to erroneous APCO vales. After the transducer was releveled to the phlebostatic axis, the APCO values were corrected.

Summary

Because of advances in technology, the use of the arterial pulse for continuous CO assessment has been refined over the past decade. The three key questions regarding a new technology have been answered. The technology was shown to be comparable to existing invasive methods of determining CO values. The physiologic principles on which the technology is based are sound and the parameters show clinical value. As the trend toward a less invasive means of monitoring patients continues, APCO provides valuable CO information, and holds promise for providing additional information that is related to the fluid status of the critically ill through the use of SVV.

Patients who might have been undermonitored before now have a means to provide information that is needed for their optimal care [5].

References

[1] Jansen JRC, van den Berg PCM. Cardiac output by thermodilution and arterial pulse contour techniques. In: Pinsky MR, Payen D, editors. Functional hemodynamic monitoring. Update in intensive care and emergency medicine, vol. 42. New York: Springer-Verlag; 2005. p. 135–52.

[2] Rhodes A, Sunderland R. Arterial pulse power analysis: the LiDCO TM plus system. In: Pinsky MR, Payen D, editors. Functional hemodynamic monitoring. Update in intensive care and emergency medicine, vol. 42. New York: Springer-Verlag; 2005. p. 183–92.

[3] Berton C, Cholley B. Equipment review: new techniques for cardiac output measurement- oesophageal Doppler, Fick principle using carbon dioxide, and pulse contour analysis. Crit Care 2002;6:216–21.

[4] Reuter DA, Goetz AE. Arterial pulse contour analysis: applicability to clinical routine. In: Pinsky MR, Payen D, editors. Functional hemodynamic monitoring. Update in intensive care and emergency medicine, vol. 42. New York: Springer-Verlag; 2005. p. 175–81.

[5] Headley JM. Pulses, pressure, and flow: emerging trends in less invasive cardiovascular monitoring. AACN News 2005;22(11):14–7.

[6] Michard F. Changes in arterial pressure during mechanical ventilation. Anesthesiology 2005;103(2): 419–28.

[7] Pinsky MR. Probing the limits of arterial pulse contour analysis to predict preload responsiveness. Anesth Analg 2003;96:1245–7.

[8] Michard F, Teboul J-L. Predicting fluid responsiveness in ICU patients: a critical analysis of the evidence. Chest 2002;121:2000–8.

[9] Parry-Jones AJD, Pittman JAL. Arterial pressure and stroke volume variability as measurements for cardiovascular optimization. International Journal of Intensive Care 2003;10(2):67–72.

[10] Guyton AC, Hall JE. Vascular distensibility and functions of the arterial and venous systems. In: Guyton AC, Hall JE, editors. Textbook of medical physiology. 10th edition. Philadelphia: Saunders; 2000. p. 152–61.

[11] Klabunde RE. Cardiac function. Cardiovascular physiology concepts. Philadelphia: Lippincott Williams & Wilkins; 2005. p. 59–90.

[12] Boulain T, Achard J-M, Teboul J-L, et al. Changes in BP induced by passive leg raising predict response to fluid loading in critically ill patients. Chest 2002; 121(4):1245–52.

[13] Lamia B, Chemla D, Richard C, et al. Clinical review: interpretation of arterial pressure wave in shock states. Crit Care 2005;9:601–6.

[14] Edwards Lifesciences, Vigileo/FloTrac Operations Manual. Irvine, California; 2005.

[15] Izzo JL, Shykoff BE. Arterial stiffness: clinical relevance, measurement, and treatment. Rev Cardiovasc Med 2001;2(1):29–40.

[16] Denault AY, Gasior TA, Gorcsan III J, et al. Determinants of aortic pressure variation during positive-pressure ventilation in man. Chest 1999;116:176–86.

[17] Manecke GR. Edwards FloTrac sensor and Vigileo monitor: easy, accurate, reliable cardiac output assessment using the arterial pulse wave. Expert Rev Med Devices 2005;2(5):523–7.

[18] Romano SM, Pistolesi M. Assessment of cardiac output from systemic arterial pressure in humans. Crit Care Med 2002;30(8):1834–41.

[19] Wesseling KH, Jansen JRC, Settels JJ, et al. Computation of aortic flow from pressure in humans using a nonlinear, three-element model. J Appl Physiol 1993; 74(5):2566–73.

[20] Available at: http://www.lidco.com. Accessed December 21, 2005.

[21] Available at:www.pulsion.com. Accessed December 21, 2005.

[22] Available at:www.edwards.com. Accessed December 21, 2005.

[23] Manecke GR, Peterson M, Auger WR. Cardiac output determination using arterial pulse: a comparison of a novel algorithm against continuous and intermittent thermodilution [abstract]. Crit Care Med 2004; 32(12);(Suppl):A43.

[24] McGee WT, Horswell J, Janvier G. Validation of a continuous cardiac output measurement using arterial pressure waveforms. Crit Care 2005;9(Suppl 1):62.

[25] Horswell J, Worley T. Continuous cardiac output measured by arterial pressure analysis in surgical patients [abstract]. Anesthiology 2005;103:A834.

[26] Gunn SR, Pinsky MR. Implications of arterial pressure variation in patients in the intensive care unit. Curr Opin Crit Care 2001;7:212–7.

[27] Safar ME, Levy BI, Struijker-Boudier H. Current perspectives on arterial stiffness and pulse pressure in hypertension and cardiovascular disease. Circulation 2003;107:2864–9.

[28] Mackenzie IS, Wilkinson IB, Cockcroft JR. Assessment of arterial stiffness in clinical practice. Q J Med 2002;95:67–74.

[29] Kuecherer HF, Just A, Kirchheim H. Evaluation of aortic compliance in humans [editorial]. Am J Physiol Heart Circ Physiol 2000;278:H1411–3.

[30] McVeigh GE, Hamilton PK, Morgan DR. Evaluation of mechanical arterial properties: clinical, experimental and therapeutic aspects. Clin Sci (Lond) 2002;102: 51–67.

[31] Vincent J-L, DeBacker D. Cardiac output measurement: is least invasive always the best? Crit Care Med 2002;30(10):2380–2.

[32] Pinsky MR. The meaning of cardiac output [editorial]. Intensive Care Med 1990;16:415–7.

[33] Wiesenack C, Fiegl C, Keyser A, et al. Continuously assessed right ventricular end-diastolic volume as a marker of cardiac preload and fluid responsiveness in mechanically ventilated cardiac surgical patients. Crit Care 2005;9:226–33.

[34] Kumar A, Anel R, Bunnell E, et al. Pulmonary artery occlusion pressure and central venous pressure fail to predict ventricular filling volume, cardiac performance, or the response to volume infusion in normal subjects. Crit Care Med 2004;32(3):691–9.

[35] Magder S. Clinical usefulness of respiratory variations in arterial pressure. Am J Respir Crit Care Med 2004; 169:151–5.

[36] Reuter DA, Kirchner A, Felbinger TW, et al. Usefulness of left ventricular stroke volume variation to assess fluid responsiveness in patients with reduced cardiac function. Crit Care Med 2003;31(5):1399–404.

[37] Perel A, Preisman S, Berkenstadt H. Arterial pressure variation during positive-pressure ventilation. In: Pinsky MR, Payen D, editors. Functional hemodynamic monitoring. Update in intensive care and emergency medicine, vol. 42. New York: Springer-Verlag; 2005. p. 313–29.

[38] Michard F, Teboul J-L. Using heart-lung interaction to assess fluid responsiveness during mechanical ventilation. Crit Care 2000;4:282–9.

[39] Kramer A, Zygun D, Hawes H, et al. Pulse pressure variation predicts fluid responsiveness following coronary artery bypass surgery. Chest 2004;126:1563–8.

ELSEVIER
SAUNDERS

Crit Care Nurs Clin N Am 18 (2006) 189–193

CRITICAL CARE
NURSING CLINICS
OF NORTH AMERICA

Esophageal Doppler Monitoring for Hemodynamic Assessment

Donna Prentice, APRN, BC, CCRN[a],*, Carrie Sona, APRN, BC, CCRN[b]

[a]Medical Intensive Care Unit, Barnes-Jewish Hospital, Mailstop 90-00-083, #1 BJH Plaza, St. Louis, MO 63110, USA
[b]Surgical/Trauma Intensive Care Unit, Barnes-Jewish Hospital, Mailstop # 90-59-346, #1 BJH Plaza, St. Louis, MO 63110, USA

The use of continuous electrocardiography, pulse oximetry, blood pressure monitoring, and capnography are the standard of care in ICUs throughout the world. The information gained from these technologies in combination with physical assessment is invaluable to clinicians but does not provide hemodynamic or, most important, blood flow information. The limitation of physical assessment when making hemodynamic decisions has been previously described [1,2]. Clinicians need additional information to assist in making critical decisions and often use hemodynamic monitoring, which includes cardiac output/index, stroke volume/index, and assessments of preload and afterload.

The pulmonary artery catheter (PAC) was developed to aid with that assessment and has been considered the clinical standard. The complexity of the PAC requires clinicians to be familiar with the operations of transducers, thermodilution cardiac output monitoring, and waveform analysis. Clinicians' knowledge of the PAC is often substandard, and it can be difficult to become and remain clinically competent [3–5]. The lack of improved outcomes associated with the PAC and overcoming the technical difficulties has resulted in some clinicians abandoning the use of the PAC [6]. Complications associated with the use of the PAC such as venous thrombosis, arrhythmias, pneumothorax, and cathe-

ter-related bloodstream infection have also been reported [7–9]. Finding a safe, reliable, and less invasive method to assist with hemodynamic and blood flow assessment is needed. The esophageal Doppler monitor (EDM) provides an alternative method of obtaining hemodynamic information.

Esophageal doppler monitoring: how does it work?

The esophageal Doppler (CardioQ, Deltex Medical, UK) uses a disposable 6-mm diameter unidirectional continuous wave Doppler transducer (4 MHz) probe. The probe is flexible yet rigid and is inserted into the midesophagus to transmit and receive an ultrasound signal (Fig. 1). The Doppler principle is based on the physical principle that the sound transmitted from the Doppler probe reflects off moving objects such as red blood cells and returns at an altered frequency [10,11]. The Doppler signal traverses the esophagus and picks up the velocity of blood flow in the descending aorta with each heartbeat. The Doppler signal also tracks the distance of the blood flow as it travels from the left ventricle. The Doppler probe is attached to a monitor to display the blood-flow velocity profile from the reflected signal. The result is an aortic waveform, with velocity on the y-axis and time on the x-axis (Fig. 2). The signal provides the clinician with information regarding contractility and preload of the left ventricle and cardiac output. The distance the blood travels down the descending thoracic aorta with each contraction is

* Corresponding author.
E-mail address: dxp7813@bjc.org (D. Prentice).

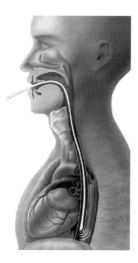

Fig. 1. EDM in the esophagus.

Table 1
Normal values for esophageal Doppler

Age (y)	Peak velocity	Flow time corrected
20	90–120 cm/s	330–360 ms
50	70–100 cm/s	330–360 ms
70	60–80 cm/s	330–360 ms

normal peak velocity is broken down into age ranges because contractility decreases with age at an estimated rate of approximately 1% per year of adult life. Low peak velocity values can reflect low contractility states.

The assessment of preload of the left ventricle is made using the length of time the blood flows from ventricle, known as flow time. The EDM corrects the flow time (FTc) to a heart rate of 60 beats per minute to allow for ease of assessment. Flow time, however, is not an absolute assessment of preload. The FTc can be low due to conditions other than volume status such as poor contractility of the left ventricle or the presence of a high afterload. The patient's FTc response can determine whether the patient requires volume or another treatment modality. If the FTc and stroke volume increase appropriately after a fluid challenge, then the patient responded to volume, and further fluid challenges may be required to optimize the preload. If the peak velocity is normal, then the FTc more accurately reflects preload. The normal values for the information obtained from the EDM are listed in Table 1. As with any hemodynamic assessment, the value of a reading at a single point in time is questionable. Following trends over time and the effects of treatment modalities allows the clinician to determine the progress of a patient.

called the stroke distance. The EDM calculates the aortic surface area using a proprietary algorithm using the patient's age, height, and weight. Using the algorithm, the EDM converts the linear measurement of stroke distance into a volumetric measurement of stroke volume. The EDM provides clinicians with a measurement of stroke volume. Stroke volume assessment provides the clinician with a way to determine the effectiveness of treatment strategies such as volume resuscitation, positive inotropic therapies, and afterload manipulations.

Cardiac output is obtained by multiplying the stroke volume by the patient's heart rate. The height at the apex of the curve—peak velocity of flow during systole—is used to assess contractility. The

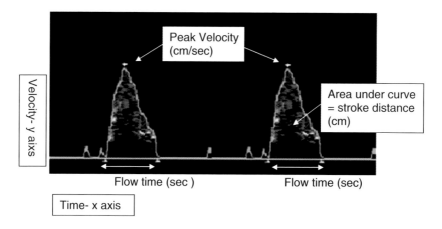

Fig. 2. Waveform components of EDM.

Obtaining hemodynamic readings

The bedside nurse can safely insert the probe within minutes, and only minor complications such as misplaced nasogastric tubes have been reported [2]. Hemodynamic readings are typically obtained quickly, allowing for early treatment interventions. The probe is lubricated and inserted into the oropharynx. Patients often require sedation to tolerate probe insertion and maintenance of the probe in the mouth to avoid biting or mouth movement that interferes with the signal [2]. The probe is inserted into the proper depth using probe markers at 35 to 40 cm from the patient's incisors based on body height (see Fig. 1). Optimizing the Doppler signal is critical to assure that the best possible data are obtained. It is important to listen to the signal and watch the waveform for analysis of proper signal acquisition. The monitor can be adjusted by the clinician to optimize the gain of the waveform and to evaluate each signal or signal average up to 20 signals. Because the Doppler signal can be intermittent, staff training is necessary to verify proper waveform analysis [12]. The ability to print the waveforms for documentation is another important consideration. Optimizing the waveform of the EDM requires the clinician to verify that (1) there is a crisp aortic sound, (2) the heart rate obtained from the EDM signal matches the heart rate from the electrocardiography monitor, (3) the arrows correctly identify the base and top of the waveforms, and (4) the green follower tracks the actual waveform without artifact (see Fig. 2).

A pneumonic can be helpful to clinicians as a reminder of the details of signal optimization (Fig. 3). Although a benefit of the EDM is that the data can be continuous, significant signal loss can occur with pa-

tients who move or with probe movement. The probe usually requires refocusing before each reading to assure that the best signal is being obtained. Refocusing the probe can be done quickly and without discomfort to the patient. Refocusing requires adjusting the height and rotation of the probe. Most patient discomfort occurs during the actual insertion. During frequent hemodynamic assessments and titration of therapy, it is best to leave the probe in place.

Limitations

The EDM is a less invasive and quicker method to aid in hemodynamic assessment of patients. As with any technology, it has limitations that clinicians must understand. One of the limitations is the size and stiffness of the probe. Although its size is similar to that of a nasogastric tube, the esophageal Doppler probe is much stiffer, limiting its use in nonintubated patients or the use of the nasopharyngeal route for insertion [13]. Most awake patients do not tolerate oropharyngeal tubes.

Another potential complication is for esophageal tissue damage. Although there have been no reports of esophageal perforation, there have been reports of significant bleeding [14]. Appropriate patient selection can minimize this risk. Insertion of the probe in patients who have significant esophageal disease (friable esophagus, esophageal tumor, significant esophageal varices with recent banding) or bleeding risk (low platelets, elevated international normalized ratio) should be avoided.

Other noted limitations are that the probe may be misplaced into the trachea, which can cause tempo-

"SHAG"
Optimal Signal Acquisition

S - loudest **S**ound...

H - **H**eart rate EDM = ECG

A - white **A**rrow s "△"accurately identify beginning, peak, and end systolic flow

G - **G**reen "Follower" envelopes waveform

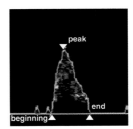

Fig. 3. Pneumonic for optimization of EDM signal.

Table 2
Esophageal Doppler monitor readings: case 1

Measurement	At probe insertion	16 h after insertion	36 h after insertion
Cardiac output/index	11.7/6.6	8.9/5.0	6.5/3.7
Peak velocity	159	122	96
Flow time corrected	355	357	442
Stroke volume	94	74	66
Systematic vascular resistance	319	503	825
Central venous pressure	11	13	13
Heart rate	124	120	98
Mean arterial pressure	58	69	80
Central venous oxygen saturation	80	78	70
Norepinephrine infusion	6 μg/min	2 μg/min	Off

rary effects on oxygenation [15]. The EDM cannot be used in patients who have coarctation of the aorta or in patients who have intra-aortic balloon pumps [11]. The lack of tissue oxygenation data is another limitation of the EDM. Clinicians can overcome this limitation by using assessment of global tissue oxygenation such as core venous oxygen saturations in conjunction with the EDM to have a more complete assessment.

Case 1

A 58-year-old unrestrained driver in a motor vehicle crash presented to the surgical/trauma ICU after a 30-minute extrication and helicopter evacuation at the scene. He had no significant past medical history. The patient suffered multisystem trauma significant for bilateral rib fractures and pneumothoraces with chest tubes, left sacroiliac pelvic fracture and symphisis pubis with diastasis, multiple thoracic and lumbar spine fractures without deficit, bladder rupture, and splenic vein laceration. The patient arrived from the operating room to the ICU intubated and sedated with central venous access and arterial line monitoring. He underwent exploratory laparotomy with repair of his ruptured bladder and splenic vein. He was volume resuscitated and stabilized. On post-injury day 5, he developed new-onset hypotension with a mean arterial blood pressure in the 50s. An

EDM was used to assist in clinical decision making and generated the information listed in Table 2.

On probe insertion, the patient was noted to have a high cardiac output, high peak velocity, high central venous oxygen saturation, and low systemic vascular resistance state. His preload assessment revealed an adequate central venous pressure and FTc. The patient was cultured to identify a source of infection. He was started on empiric antibiotics. A norepinephrine infusion was started and titrated for a mean arterial pressure of greater than 65. Bronchoscopic alveolar lavage culture results were positive for *Pseudomonas aeruginosa*, and antibiotic therapy was tailored for the specific sensitivities. The patient responded appropriately to therapy for sepsis, and his response with normalizing systemic vascular resistance and cardiac output was easily monitored with the EDM.

Case 2

A 31-year-old woman was admitted to the medical ICU with hypotension and respiratory failure. She had past medical history of type 2 diabetes mellitus and hypertension. The EDM probe was placed at 8:00 AM to help assess the reason for her hypotension. The EDM readings are listed in Table 3. She was begun on dobutamine at 8:30 AM, with repeat vital signs and EDM readings at 9:30 AM and 10:30 AM as the dobutamine was titrated up. The trend of the EDM allowed the clinician to see the effectiveness of the positive inotropic therapy. She became less tachycardic, with dramatic improvements in her cardiac output, stoke volume, peak velocity, and flow time. Little to no change was noted

Table 3
Esophageal Doppler monitor readings: case 2

Measurement	Time		
	8:00 AM	9:30 AM	10:30 AM
Blood pressure	91/60	95/63	91/59
Pulse	130	102	100
Respiratory rate	26	12	12
Cardiac output/index	1.7/0.8	4.6/2.1	6.3/2.9
Stroke volume	13	45	60
Peak velocity	35	62.5	83.5
Flow time corrected	241	348	363
Central venous pressure	16	12	8
Dobutamine dose	—	2.5 μg/kg/min	5 μg/kg/min

Table 4
Comparison of hemodynamic data and shock states

	Pulmonary artery catheter		Esophageal Doppler		
Type of shock	Central venous pressure	Pulmonary capillary wedge pressure (PCWP)	Cardiac output	Flow time corrected	Peak velocity
Hypovolemia	↓	↓	↓	↓	Normal or ↓ in extreme hypovolemia
Cardiogenic shock (left ventricular failure)	↑ or normal	↑	↓	↓	↓↓
Low systemic vascular resistance (distributive)	Normal or ↓	Normal or ↓	↑	Normal or ↑	Normal or ↑
Obstructive (cardiac tamponade)	↑ (= with PCWP)	↑ (= with central venous pressure)	↓	↓	↓

in her blood pressure, representing the poor reflection of blood pressure on measuring blood flow.

Summary

The EDM is a less invasive and clinically useful tool to obtain hemodynamic information. This information is clinically relevant and important in guiding therapies for critically ill patients. The bedside clinician must understand the importance of proper signal acquisition and how to optimize and interpret the hemodynamic information obtained from the EDM (Table 4). It is also important to understand appropriate indications for and limitations of the EDM.

References

[1] Eisenberg PR, Jaffe AS, Schuster DP. Clinical evaluation compared to pulmonary artery catheterization in the hemodynamic assessment of critically ill patients. Crit Care Med 1984;12:549–53.

[2] Iregui MG, Prentice D, Sherman G, et al. Physicians' estimates of cardiac index and intravascular volume based on clinical assessment versus transesophageal Doppler measurement obtained by critical care nurses. Am J Crit Care 2003;12:336–42.

[3] Iberti TJ, Dailey EK, Leibowitz AB, et al. Assessment of critical care nurses' knowledge of the pulmonary artery catheter. The pulmonary artery catheter study group. Crit Care Med 1994;22:1674–8.

[4] Iberti TJ, Fischer EP, Leibowitz AB, et al. A multi-

center study of physicians' knowledge of the pulmonary artery catheter. JAMA 1990;264:2928–32.

[5] Gnaegi A, Feihl F, Perret C. Intensive care physicians' insufficient knowledge of right heart catheterization at the bedside: time to act? Crit Care Med 1997;25:213–20.

[6] Connors Jr AF, Speroff T, Dawson NV, et al. The effectiveness of right heart catheterization in the initial care of critically ill patients. JAMA 1996;276:889–97.

[7] Prentice D, Ahrens T. Controversies in the use of the pulmonary artery catheter. J Cardiovasc Nurs 2001; 15(2):1–5.

[8] Ivanov R, Allen J, Calvin JE. The incidence of major morbidity in critically ill patients managed with pulmonary artery catheters: a meta analysis. Crit Care Med 2000;28:615–9.

[9] Kelso LA. Complications associated with pulmonary artery catheterization. New Horizons 1997;5:259–63.

[10] Ott K, Johnson D, Ahrens T. New technologies in the assessment of hemodynamic parameters. J Cardiovascular Nurs 2001;15(2):41–55.

[11] Turner M. Doppler-based hemodynamic monitoring. AACN Clin Issues 2003;14(2):220–31.

[12] LeFant JY, Bruelle P, Aya AGM, et al. Training is required to improve the reliability of esophageal Doppler to measure cardiac output in critically ill patients. Intensive Care Med 1998;24:347–52.

[13] Atlas G, Mort T. Placement of the esophageal Doppler ultrasound probe in awake patients. Chest 2001; 119:319.

[14] St-Pierre J, Fortier LP, Couture P, et al. Massive gastrointestinal hemorrhage after transesophageal echocardiography probe insertion. Can J Anesth 1998; 45(12):1196–9.

[15] Ortega R, Hesselvik JF, Chandhok D, et al. When the transesophageal echo probe goes into the trachea. J Cardiothorac Vasc Anesth 1999;13(1):114–5.

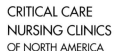

CRITICAL CARE
NURSING CLINICS
OF NORTH AMERICA

Crit Care Nurs Clin N Am 18 (2006) 195 – 202

Bioimpedance Cardiography Measurements of Cardiac Output and Other Cardiovascular Parameters

Nancy M. Albert, PhD, CCNS, CCRN, CNA

Cleveland Clinic, 9500 Euclid Avenue, P-32, Cleveland, OH 44195, USA

Impedance cardiography was first proposed by Kubicek and colleagues [1] for measurement of stroke volume, cardiac output, and other cardiovascular parameters for aerospace programs [2]. Since that time, software refinements and technical improvements in bioimpedance measurement methods that are used in determining left ventricular ejection time, change in impedance with systole, and other markers of systole and diastole provide greater accuracy of noninvasive hemodynamic data.

Impedance cardiography increased in popularity in the United States in the late 1990s and early 2000s for three main reasons: (1) the use of pulmonary artery catheters decreased after researchers reported that they were associated with increased hospital morbidity (pulmonary embolism, infection, bleeding, and pulmonary artery rupture) and mortality [3,4], and the Society of Critical Care Medicine developed a consensus statement about using these catheters in patients who have a variety of diseases and disorders [5]; (2) thoracic bioimpedance method by one company (Cardiodynamics International, San Diego, California) was widely available and found to be accurate for many patient populations; most notably, after open heart surgery [6,7], chronic heart failure [8,9], and when mechanically ventilated [10]; and (3) research results demonstrated the value of non-invasive impedance cardiography data in a variety of clinical settings, including hospital, ambulatory, and specialty care (ie, atrioventricular optimization during

left ventricular permanent pacing [11]), and for a variety of purposes, including diagnosis, assessment, prognosis determination, and management.

Not all bioimpedance cardiography systems are alike. The algorithm that is used to determine baseline bioimpedance during diastole and changes in impedance during systole vary by company, although they may be modifications of a popular algorithm that was developed to measure aortic stroke volume by means of its impedance change. Additionally, system type (whole-body or thoracic bioimpedance cardiography) and the methods that are used to collect data are not consistent between manufacturers. Thus, it cannot be assumed that one system is equal to another. It is important for nurses who use this technology to be vigilant about reviewing the available research that is associated with the device being used to ensure that bioimpedance cardiography data accurately reflect data that are collected by traditional (invasive cardiac output) techniques. Vigilance includes reviewing published research results from peer-reviewed journals as it relates to the patient population of interest. Not all devices have been tested for accuracy and reliability in similar patient populations. Devices may be housed to appear similar, but it is not acceptable to believe that two systems by two manufacturers work similarly and provide similar result accuracy. This paper describes impedance technique and device types, discusses available hemodynamic data parameters, discusses differences between impedance cardiography and data that are derived from invasive pulmonary artery catheters, and explains how nurses can apply bioimpedance cardiography in a variety of patient populations.

E-mail address: albertn@ccf.org

doi:10.1016/j.ccell.2006.01.008

Impedance technique and device types

Bioimpedance cardiography is based on measurements of impedance (or resistance) to transmission of a small electrical current throughout the body (whole-body bioimpedance) or chest area (thoracic bioimpedance). In the body, electrical current passes through conduits of high and low conductance. Conduits of low impedance (lowest resistance, equals high conductance) are blood (150 Ω/cm) and plasma (63 Ω/cm). Resistance of electrical current is higher (lower conductance) for cardiac muscle (750 Ω/cm); lungs, reflecting air (1275 Ω/cm); and fat (2500 Ω/cm) [12]. Thus, when alternating low-level electrical current is applied to the whole body or thoracic area, the primary distribution is to the blood and extracellular fluid. Changes in the body's resistance to electrical current flow over time (in milliseconds) are associated with dynamic changes in the blood and plasma. As the aortic valve opens and blood is ejected swiftly into the aorta and the arterial branches, impedance to electrical current flow is decreased. During diastole, impedance to electrical flow returns to baseline. In the capillaries and venous system, blood volume is mostly constant because these vessels are nonpulsatile. Therefore, the changes in impedance that are noted by a thoracic bioimpedance cardiography device reflect an increase in aortic pressure during systole, whereas changes in whole-body impedance reflect a proportional increase in the measurable conductance of the whole body during systole [12].

Whole-body bioimpedance devices

To collect patient signals, these systems usually use two pairs of proprietary electrodes that inject (transmit) current (placed just proximal to the wrists and ankles on the internal side), and another pair of electrodes that sense (receive) baseline and changes in impedance (placed approximately 5 cm proximal to the injecting electrodes). In patients who have severe peripheral edema or severe peripheral vascular disease, electrodes may be placed higher up on the lower leg; if a venous graft wound is present (ie, when a vein is harvested for coronary artery bypass grafting) the lateral side of the ankles can be used [13].

Thoracic bioimpedance devices

In these devices, manufacturers may use one or two pairs of injecting and sensing electrodes to meet their needs. When the system calls for one injecting and one sensing electrode, they often are placed at the left base of the neck and along the xiphoid process, respectively [14]. When the system calls for two pairs of electrodes, the sensing and injecting electrodes are placed 180° apart (opposite sides) at the base of the neck (sensing electrodes are proximal to injecting electrodes) and at the midaxillary line at the level of the xiphoid process [15]. In both systems, the electrodes mark the upper and lower limits of the thorax.

Although all systems require injecting and sensing electrodes to measure bioimpedance and calculate stroke volume, differences between device manufacturers abound. In some systems, the placement of electrodes is critical to receiving accurate hemodynamic data, whereas in others, electrode placement is less critical and can be done by an untrained operator. Some systems require separate ECG electrodes to measure pulse rate and obtain ECG data; other systems collect ECG data through the two pairs of electrodes that already are placed for bioimpedance data collection.

Hemodynamic data

Hemodynamic data is obtained by two methods: parameters that are measured directly from data obtained from the sensing and ECG electrodes and parameters that are calculated from measured data. The injecting electrodes deliver low-amperage, high-frequency (30 kHz, 1.4 mA to 75 kHz, 1.8 mA; varies by manufacturer) alternating current through the whole-body or thorax, and the sensing electrodes detect baseline bioimpedance (during diastole, when aortic blood volume decreases) and changes in bioimpedance (at the beginning of each systole as aortic blood volume increases [maximum impedance gradient]) with each cardiac cycle. In addition, systems measure a third variable: ventricular ejection time so that stroke volume can be calculated. Examples of measured and calculated parameters are listed in Table 1. Normal values are not included because these vary slightly by manufacturer.

Parameters that are available through bioimpedance cardiography do not mimic data that are obtained by pulmonary artery catheter (Table 2). Of most importance are the unavailability of right atrial and pulmonary artery wedge pressure (PAWP) values and the availability of contractility parameters through bioimpedance data. The significance of each is described below.

Table 1
An example of measured and calculated parameters derived from a bioimpedance cardiography system

Measured parameters	Calculated parameters
Thoracic or whole-body fluid content (intravascular and extravascular volume)	Stroke volume/stroke index
Heart rate	Cardiac output/cardiac index
Acceleration index	Systemic vascular resistance/ systemic vascular resistance
Velocity index	Left cardiac work/left cardiac work index
Pre-ejection period	Systolic time ratio
Left ventricular ejection time	

Right atrial pressure can be obtained and entered into the bioimpedance device by palpating the right internal jugular vein for elevated pressure and using a formula to change cm H_2O pressure into mm Hg (divide cm H_2O measurement by 1.36 to derive mm Hg value). Although elevated jugular venous pressure is a surrogate for elevated right atrial pressure values, in one study, only 63% of patients who had New York Heart Association (NYHA) functional class III–IV symptoms and advanced heart failure had an elevated jugular venous pressure when hospitalized [16]. As a marker for obtaining right atrial pressure data, right jugular venous pressure has good specificity but less than adequate sensitivity. When present, an elevated jugular venous pressure was associated with an increased risk for death or hospitalization for heart failure and death from pump failure [16]. As a hemodynamic parameter, right atrial pressure availability is valuable to clinicians for diagnosis, assessment, and management. In addition, right atrial pressure data are necessary to calculate systemic vascular resistance/ index. When a default or inaccurate right atrial pressure value is entered into the bioimpedance system, systemic vascular resistance data do not reflect actual patient values. The level of inaccuracy may not prevent using the data to monitor changes in systemic vascular resistance over time, especially when making changes in pharmacologic therapies that are known to affect this parameter in patients who have hypertension and chronic heart failure.

There is no reliable equivalent to obtaining PAWP values. Two studies found that B-type natriuretic peptide (BNP) values correlated with PAWP values in patients who had decompensated chronic heart failure who received care in an ICU with invasive hemodynamic monitoring; PAWP and BNP values decreased with therapy [17,18]. However, when serial BNP measurements were compared with invasively derived data in a study of 39 patients who had severe heart failure, there was no correlation between BNP and any hemodynamically derived variable over a 36-hour period even though a decrease was noted in PAWP and BNP from baseline to 12 hours of therapy. A change in BNP was not associated with a change in PAWP in any of the patients [19].

Researchers have tried to correlate PAWP to thoracic fluid content index, an impedance cardiography variable that is described in Table 2. In a study that directly compared PAWP readings with thoracic fluid content index data that were collected at the same time, correlation was r = 0.05 (P = .71) [9]. In another study that used similar methodology, researchers converted thoracic fluid content index and PAWP values into quartiles to reflect hypovolemia, normal volume, moderate hypervolemia, and severe hypervolemia. In addition, quartile values for thoracic fluid content index were specified for men and women. There was a moderate positive correlation between thoracic fluid content index and PAWP (r = 0.39; P = .025); however, researchers did not believe that the correlation was strong enough to allow for clinical decision making without further study [8].

PAWP data are needed to calculate pulmonary vascular resistance/index. For some patient populations, the need for PAWP or pulmonary vascular resistance/index data might be arbitrary; however, in patients who have advanced chronic heart failure, PAWP value while hospitalized was associated with survival after hospital discharge, functional status, and freedom from symptoms, and was considered to be a more important variable than cardiac output [20,21]. Additionally, PAWP is associated directly with left ventricular end-diastolic pressure and volume. Using PAWP to monitor improvement in volume and congestion in patients who have advanced or recently decompensated heart failure can be beneficial. Freedom from congestion predicted good survival in patients who were discharged from the hospital after NYHA functional class IV symptoms [22]. The inability to receive systemic vascular resistance data (when right atrial pressure data is unavailable), compounded with the lack of PAWP data (or an equivalent), could minimize the benefits of bioimpedance cardiography monitoring depending on the setting, purpose for monitoring, and patient population.

An advantage to bioimpedance cardiography monitoring is the ability to obtain specific indices of left ventricular contractility that are not available with a pulmonary artery catheter (see Table 2 for

Table 2
Hemodynamic data

Impedance cardiography	Pulmonary artery catheter
Stroke volume/stroke index	Stroke volume/stroke index
Cardiac output/cardiac index	Cardiac output/cardiac index
Systemic vascular resistance/systemic vascular resistance	Systemic vascular resistance/systemic vascular resistance index
Not available	Pulmonary vascular resistance/pulmonary vascular resistance index
Left cardiac and stroke work/left cardiac and stroke work index	Left cardiac and stroke work/left cardiac and stroke work index
Not available	Pulmonary capillary wedge pressure
Not available	Right atrial pressure
Other contractility parameters:	
Systolic time ratio: the ratio of electrical to mechanical systole. Provides data on electro-mechanical heart performance; as heart failure worsens the ratio of electrical to mechanical systole becomes higher.	Not available
Pre-ejection period: the time interval from the beginning of electrical stimulation of the ventricles to the opening of the aortic valve. Reflects isovolumetric contraction phase of systole.	
Left ventricular ejection time: Time measured from the opening to the closing of the aortic valve; represents mechanical systole.	
Velocity index: represents the peak velocity of blood flow in the aorta. In patients who have heart failure, this parameter may remain in the normal range, even though the acceleration contractility index is reduced.	
Acceleration index: The initial acceleration of blood flow in the aorta; occurs within the first 10–20 milliseconds after the aortic valve opens. The stronger the ventricle contracts, the higher the value; measured in seconds squared.	
Thoracic fluid content: represents the electrical conductivity of the chest cavity (requires a thoracic bioimpedance cardiography device to obtain this data); determined by intravascular, intra-alveolar, and extravascular (interstitial) fluids in the thorax. Uses impedance data and divides it by 1. Thus, high impedance = less thoracic volume = low thoracic fluid content. Low impedance = more thoracic volume (because electrical current has less resistance to changes in blood and plasma versus air) = high thoracic fluid content.	Not available

terms and definitions). In patients who have advanced, chronic heart failure, the availability of specific contractility parameters provides additional data for determining worsening of left ventricular function and prognosis (major heart failure events and mortality).

Impedance cardiography was used to predict the occurrence of major heart failure events. In the PRospective Evaluation of cardiac Decompensation in patients with heart failure by Impedance Cardiography Test (PREDICT) multicenter trial, researchers wanted to learn if noninvasive thoracic impedance cardiography parameters could predict short-term risk, defined as all-cause death or emergency depart-

ment visit or hospitalization due to worsening heart failure. Data were collected every 2 weeks for 26 weeks in 212 patients. Twenty-nine percent of all subjects had events. When impedance cardiography data, vital signs, baseline characteristics, and a visual analog scale of how patients felt at the time of each office visit on a scale of 1 to 100 were analyzed, important variables that preceded an event were identified. These varaibles included lower self-rating on the visual analog scale, higher NYHA functional class, lower systolic blood pressure, and three impedance cardiography parameters: lower velocity index, higher thoracic fluid content index, and diminished left ventricular ejection time. When the three impedance cardiography variables were combined and compared with other statistically significant variables that preceded a heart failure event, the composite impedance cardiography score had the strongest association for a subsequent heart failure event [23]. Therefore, when combined with other variables—especially visual analog scale, NYHA functional class, and systolic blood pressure—impedance cardiography can identify patients with advanced heart failure who are at the highest and lowest risk for a heart failure event.

Impedance cardiography contractility parameters provide objective data in chronic heart failure that are related to changes in functional status and prognosis. In a study of 64 ambulatory patients, baseline data were compared with data at 3 months. Changes in stroke index, left ventricular ejection time, and systolic time ratio correlated significantly with changes in NYHA functional class, 6-minute walk distance, patient visual analog scale score, and quality of life score using the Minnesota Living with Heart Failure Questionnaire [24]. Another group of researchers used systolic time ratio to predict mortality in ambulatory patients who had advanced heart failure. A greater systolic time ratio reflected a longer pre-ejection period (isovolumetric contraction), diminished left ventricular ejection time, or both and was associated with worsening left ventricular function. In this study, 78% of patients that expired had an elevated systolic time ratio compared with 60% of patients who survived ($P<.007$). Researchers concluded that elevation of systolic time ratio correlated with NYHA functional class and mortality when reviewed as an isolated parameter, and that it may be useful in risk stratification and management of outpatients who have heart failure [25].

After cardiac transplantation, acute rejection is a main complication that requires early identification and treatment. Researchers used thoracic bioimpedance in 35 patients who had undergone heart transplants to determine if hemodynamic parameters would predict acute rejection at the time of endomyocardial biopsy. The acceleration index was significantly lower in patients who had acute rejection episodes than in patients who had normal biopsies [26]. As a diagnostic parameter, acceleration index is an early indicator of failing left ventricular contractility; it decreases before stroke volume does. In this study, the sensitivity was 71% and the specificity was 100%. Thus, bioimpedance cardiography was a quick and noninvasive technique that identified worsening contractility. It could be used in between routinely ordered invasive procedures at ambulatory follow-up visits.

Therapeutic value of impedance cardiography

Resistant hypertension

Failure to achieve an adequate response to antihypertensive therapy is a burden to clinicians. In a hospital or ambulatory setting, aggressive treatment of resistant hypertension can be individualized when serial hemodynamic measurements beyond blood pressure values are available to the health care team. Specific classes of drugs may work better in hypertensive patients who respond with elevated systemic vascular resistance versus increased cardiac output. Angiotensin-converting enzyme inhibitors, angiotensin receptor blockers, thiazide diuretics, β-blockers, and calcium channel blockers have different effects on cardiac output, total peripheral resistance, systemic vascular resistance, and plasma volume that can lead to transient symptomatic hypotension and fatigue [27]. When new drugs are added and used in combination, precise tracking of hemodynamic measurements can prompt corrections in hemodynamic abnormalities and facilitate optimum drug use and dosing. An intensive treatment program was set up for 3 months in 104 patients who had resistant hypertension. Drug selection was based on hemodynamic data and a predefined algorithm or a hypertension specialist's medical opinion. Taler and colleagues [28] found that both treatment groups had lowered blood pressure in 3 months, but that the serial hemodynamic measurement/drug selection with algorithm group was more likely to have a blood pressure less than 140/90 mm Hg (56% versus 33%; $P<.05$). The impedance cardiography hemodynamic monitoring/drugs by algorithm arm of Taler and colleagues' trial was replicated by community physicians in a case series of 21 patients who had uncontrolled blood pressure and were taking two agents. Researchers enhanced pharmacologic decision making when guided by impedance cardiography [29].

Psychologic mood states have been believed to influence hemodynamic responses. Impedance-derived variables and the profile of mood states (POMS) were measured in 71 normotensive and hypertensive individuals to determine relationships. Participants with high tension–anxiety by POMS had lower stroke volume, and those with higher fatigue-inertia POMS had lower cardiac output and higher total peripheral vascular resistance [30]. There was no association between POMS, heart rate, and blood pressure or between POMS anger-hostility and hemodynamic variables, even though older research showed that high anger or hostility increased blood pressure. Researchers concluded that mood states were associated with hemodynamic variables that underlie blood pressure and that stroke volume, cardiac output, and total peripheral resistance may be more sensitive to subtle differences in mood than are heart rate and blood pressure.

Pacemaker

After pacemaker insertion, changes in cardiac function can cause suboptimal timing of the atrioventricular (AV) interval during AV sequential (dual chamber right ventricular and biventricular) pacing, which lead to changes in left ventricular preload that reduce systolic performance. Doppler echocardiography is an established method to optimize AV interval; however it is costly, time-consuming, and operator dependent. Because it is expected that hemodynamic measurements are altered with suboptimal AV interval timing, using impedance cardiography to optimize the AV interval offers a simple, cost-effective solution. Researchers found that impedance cardiography was a useful hemodynamic monitoring technology for AV optimization in acute atrioventricular pacing with temporary wires in refractory patients who had heart failure [31,32], in biventricular pacemaker follow-up when patients were programmed with synchronous right and left ventricular pacing [33–35], and during permanent left ventricular pacing [11]. In most studies, impedance cardiography was compared with quantitative tissue Doppler echocardiography and was found to be precise ($r=0.67-0.844$).

Heart failure

Most research on the value of impedance cardiography was conducted in patients who had heart failure, because it represents a costly, debilitating medical condition with abnormal hemodynamics. In addition to using impedance cardiography to predict future events (PREDICT trial), prognosis, and heart failure diagnosis, clinicians used impedance cardiography to aid in decision making when initiating and titrating intravenous agents that prompt changes in hemodynamics [36,37], when weaning patients from intermittent infusion therapy [38], and when transitioning patients from intravenous inotropic to intravenous vasodilator therapy [39]. In these situations, the additional hemodynamic information was useful in tailoring therapies to individual patients. Current intravenous agents that alter hemodynamics (nesiritide, dobutamine, milrinone) are not advocated for outpatient intermittent infusion; however, noninvasive trending of cardiac output and other hemodynamic variables can provide prognostic information that aids in decision making about end-of-life care that might include use of these therapies. In addition, hemodynamic monitoring may assist clinicians in learning how to optimize newer intravenous agents that alter contractility (ie, calcium sensitizers) or neuroendocrine activation (ie, vasopressin antagonists), once approved for use in acute decompensation.

Other patient populations

Because impedance cardiography assesses dynamic changes in blood and plasma, it can be used as an alternative to invasive hemodynamic monitoring in many settings beyond traditional critical care or anesthesia and in many patient populations. Recurrent intradialytic hypotension causes patient discomfort and clinician interface in patients who require acute or chronic hemodialysis. Using impedance cardiography, researchers found that patients who experienced symptomatic hypotension during dialysis had a greater decline in blood volume and cardiac output than did stable patients. The real issue was that these patients had a significant decrease in systemic vascular resistance when compared with stable patients who had an increase in systemic vascular resistance [40]. Using this information, impedance cardiography monitoring can be used during dialysis treatments, as a means of assessing the usefulness of prevention or control interventions, in patients who are known to have recurrent intradialytic hypotension.

In peripartum women who have preeclampsia, thoracic fluid content monitoring may provide benefits beyond monitoring of cardiac output and vasoconstriction. Impedance cardiography monitoring was used to measure thoracic fluid content in 134 peripartum women in uncomplicated early labor (n=72), with preeclampsia (n=50) or in pulmonary edema (n=12). Women who had peripartum pulmonary edema had significantly higher thoracic fluid content by impedance cardiography than did those who had mild or severe preeclampsia. A thoracic fluid content of at least 65 kΩ was associated with peripartum pulmonary edema (sensitivity 83.3%, specificity 86.9%, negative predictive value of 98.1%). Using this information, thoracic fluid content monitoring may lead to medical intervention in peripartum women who have preeclampsia, even when overt clinical symptoms are absent [41].

In chronic fatigue syndrome, the cause is unknown but there is accumulating evidence of a problem with circulation. Thus, researchers used impedance cardiography to measure cardiac output and assess its relationship to presenting symptoms.

Impedance cardiography findings in 38 patients who had mild (n=20) or severe (n=18) illness were compared with 27 matched, sedentary control subjects. Patients who had severe chronic fatigue syndrome had significantly lower stroke volume and cardiac output than did control subjects and less severely ill patients, which provided a preliminary indication of reduced circulation [42]. Using this information, methods to improve circulatory insufficiency could be targeted in patients who have severe symptoms from chronic fatigue syndrome. Regular impedance cardiography monitoring could provide evidence of therapy effectiveness, and may aid in future treatment modalities and clinical implications.

As described above in three studies of different patient populations, monitoring changes in circulation and hemodynamic status may play an important role in advancing science and patient management. Impedance cardiography is a feasible method for continuous or intermittent noninvasive hemodynamic assessment of patients. In settings that use bolus thermodilution method as a standard of care (especially critical care and anesthesia), bias and precision between hemodynamic data collection methods in specific patient populations must be assured. In many patient settings (especially emergency and outpatient care), health care providers do not rely on invasive hemodynamic monitoring in clinical assessment and decision making; however, patients may benefit from one-time or regular monitoring of impedance cardiography hemodynamics as an adjunct in guiding medical therapy, determining therapeutic intervention effectiveness, and aiding in prognosis determination.

Summary

Validation studies that correlate well with standard thermodilution techniques and data that report the usefulness of noninvasive technology in providing unbiased hemodynamic information in a variety of patient populations and clinical settings should prompt nurses to consider impedance cardiography as an adjunct to, or possibly as a replacement for standard invasive hemodynamic monitoring techniques. Hemodynamic data that are provided in impedance cardiography systems are not directly equivalent to those of a pulmonary artery catheter. Impedance cardiography provides contractility data that can augment traditional hemodynamic information. Current systems measure whole-body or thoracic impedance to electrical current, and are user friendly, easy to apply, and safe. The use of impedance cardiography may augment the relationships between hemodynamic parameters and cardiovascular and circulation disorders that may prompt or advance patient care.

References

[1] Kubicek WG, Karnegis JN, Patterson RP, et al. Development and evaluation of an impedance cardiac output system. Aerosp Med 1966;37:1208–12.
[2] Kubicek WG, Patterson RP, Witsoe DA. Impedance cardiography as a noninvasive method of monitoring cardiac function and other parameters of the cardiovascular system. Ann N Y Acad Sci 1970;170:724–32.
[3] Connors AF, Speroff T, Dawson NV, et al. The effectiveness of right heart catheterization in the initial care of critically ill patients. SUPPORT Investigators. JAMA 1996;276:889–97.
[4] Sandham JD, Hull RD, Brant RF, et al. A randomized, controlled trial of the use of pulmonary-artery catheters in high-risk surgical patients. N Engl J Med 2003;348:5–14.
[5] Pulmonary Artery Catheter Consensus Conference participants. Pulmonary artery catheter consensus conference: consensus statement. Crit Care Med 1997;25:910–25.
[6] Sageman WS, Riffenburgh RH, Spiess BD, et al. Equivalence of bioimpedance and thermodilution in measuring cardiac index after cardiac surgery. J Cardiothor Vasc Anesthesia 2002;16:8–14.
[7] Van De Water JM, Miller TW, Vogel RL, et al. Impedance cardiography: the next vital sign technology? Chest 2003;123:2028–33.
[8] Albert NM, Hail MD, Li J, et al. Equivalence of the bioimpedance and thermodilution methods in measuring cardiac output in hospitalized patients with advanced, decompensated chronic heart failure. Am J Crit Care 2004;13:469–79.
[9] Drazner MH, Thompson B, Rosenberg PB, et al. Comparison of impedance cardiography with invasive hemodynamic measurements in patients with heart failure secondary to ischemic or nonischemic cardiomyopathy. Am J Cardiol 2002;89:993–5.
[10] Ziegler D, Grotti L, Krucke G. Comparison of cardiac output measurements by TEB vs. intermittent bolus thermodilution in mechanical ventilated patients. Chest 1999;116(Suppl 2):281S.
[11] Tse HF, Yu C, Park E, et al. Impedance cardiography for atrioventricular interval optimization during permanent left ventricular pacing. Pacing Clin Electrophysiol 2003;26(Pt. II):189–91.
[12] Cotter G, Moshkovitz Y, Kaluski E, et al. Accurate, noninvasive continuous monitoring of cardiac output by whole-body electrical impedance. Chest 2004;125:1431–40.
[13] Kaukinen S, Kööbi T, Bi Y, et al. Cardiac output measurement after coronary artery bypass grafting using bolus thermodilution, continuous thermodilution, and

whole-body impedance cardiography. J Cardiothorac Vasc Anesth 2003;17:199–203.

[14] Tordi N, Mourot L, Matusheski N, et al. Measurements of cardiac output during constant exercises: comparison of two non-invasive techniques. Int J Sports Med 2004;25:145–9.

[15] Lasater M, Von Rueden KT. Outpatient cardiovascular management utilizing impedance cardiography. AACN Clin Issues 2003;14:240–50.

[16] Drazner MH, Rame JE, Stevenson LW, et al. Prognostic importance of elevated jugular venous pressure and a third heart sound in patients with heart failure. N Engl J Med 2001;345:574–81.

[17] Kazanegra R, Cheng V, Garcia A, et al. A rapid test for B-type natriuretic peptide correlates with falling wedge pressures in patients treated for decompensated heart failure: a pilot study. J Card Fail 2001;7:21–9.

[18] Johnson W, Omland T, Hall C, et al. Neurohormonal activation rapidly decreases after intravenous therapy with diuretics and vasodilators for class IV heart failure. J Am Coll Cardiol 2002;39:1623–9.

[19] O'Neill JO, Bott-Silverman CE, McRae AT, et al. B-type natriuretic peptide levels are not a surrogate marker for invasive hemodynamics during management of patients with severe heart failure. Am Heart J 2005;149:363–9.

[20] Steimle AE, Stevenson LW, Chelimsky-Fallick C, et al. Sustained hemodynamic efficacy of therapy tailored to reduce filling pressures in survivors with advanced heart failure. Circulation 1997;96:1165–72.

[21] Shah MR, Stinnett SS, McNulty SE, et al. Hemodynamics as surrogate end points for survival in advanced heart failure: an analysis from FIRST. Am Heart J 2001;141:908–14.

[22] Lucas C, Johnson W, Hamilton MA, et al. Freedom from congestion predicts good survival despite class IV symptoms of heart failure. Am Heart J 2000;140:840–7.

[23] Abraham W, Trupp R, Mehra MR, et al. A multivariate impedance cardiography composite score can predict the occurrence of major heart failure events: the PREDICT study. Circulation 2004;110(Suppl III):597.

[24] Vijayaraghavan K, Crum S, Cherukuri S, et al. Association of impedance cardiography parameters with changes in functional and quality-of-life measures in patients with chronic heart failure. Congest Heart Fail 2004;10(Suppl 2):22–7.

[25] Zewail A, Eastwood C, Scroggins N, et al. Use of systolic time ration and B-type natriuretic peptide to predict mortality in patients with heart failure. J Card Fail 2003;9(Suppl):S105.

[26] Weinhold C, Reichenspurner H, Fülle P, et al. Registration of thoracic electrical bioimpedance for early diagnosis of rejection after heart transplantation. J Heart Lung Transplant 1993;12:832–6.

[27] Taler SJ, Augustine JE, Textor SC. A hemodynamic approach to resistant hypertension. Cong Heart Fail 2000;6(2):90–3.

[28] Taler SJ, Textor SC, Augustine J. Resistant hypertension comparing hemodynamic management to specialist care. Hypertension 2002;39:982–8.

[29] Sharman D, Gomes C, Rutherford J. Improvement in blood pressure control with impedance cardiography guided pharmacologic decision making. Cong Heart Fail 2004;10:54–8.

[30] Yu BH, Nelesen R, Ziegler MG, et al. Mood states and impedance cardiography-derived hemodynamics. Ann Behav Med 2001;23(1):21–5.

[31] Johnson WB, Voegtlin L, Bailin SJ, et al. Impedance cardiography for acute pacing AV optimization. J Card Fail 2001;7(Suppl 2):52.

[32] Hayes DL, Hayes SN, Hyberger LK. Atrioventricular interval optimization technique: impedance measurements vs. echo/Doppler. Pacing Clin Electrophysiol 1998;21(4):969.

[33] Hayes DL, Hayes SN, Hyberger LK, et al. Atrioventricular interval optimization after biventricular pacing: echo/Doppler vs. impedance plethysmography. Pacing Clin Electrophysiol 2000;23(4):590.

[34] Santos JF, Parreira L, Madeira J, et al. Noninvasive hemodynamic monitorization for AV interval optimization in patients with ventricular resynchronization therapy. Rev Port Cardiol 2003;22(9):1091–8.

[35] Adachi H, Hiratsuji T, Sakurai S, et al. Impedance cardiography and quantitative tissue Doppler echocardiography for evaluating the effect of cardiac resynchronization therapy: a case report. J Cardiol 2003;42(1):37–42.

[36] Summers RL, Parrott CW, Quale C, et al. Use of noninvasive hemodynamics to aid decision making in the initiation and titration of neurohormonal agents. Cong Heart Fail 2004;10(Suppl 2):28–31.

[37] Mulki G, Pisano C, Gallagher C, et al. Safety and efficacy of intermittent, short-term, outpatient nesiritide infusions for the treatment of decompensated heart failure. J Card Fail 2003;9(Suppl):S68.

[38] Choudhary G, Fayn E, Vrushab R, et al. Intermittent milrinone and beta blocker therapy: hemodynamic indicators of successful weaning from inotropes. J Card Fail 2000;6(3):73.

[39] Squiers J, Vora K. Results from a pilot study to determine the feasibility in transitioning outpatient CHF patients from intermittent intravenous inotrope therapy to nesiritide. J Card Fail 2003;9(Suppl):S90.

[40] Roggekamp SB, de Vries PM, ter Wee PM. Systemic vascular resistance in intradialytic hypotension determined by means of impedance cardiography. Blood Purif 1998;16:281–9.

[41] Newman R, Pierre H, Scardo J. Thoracic fluid conductivity in peripartum women with pulmonary edema. Obstet Gynaecol 1999;94:48–51.

[42] Peckerman A, Lamanca JJ, Dahl KA, et al. Abnormal impedance cardiography predicts symptom severity in chronic fatigue syndrome. Am J Med Sci 2003;326(2):55–60.

ELSEVIER
SAUNDERS

Crit Care Nurs Clin N Am 18 (2006) 203 – 209

CRITICAL CARE
NURSING CLINICS
OF NORTH AMERICA

Continuous Central Venous Oximetry Monitoring

Cindy Goodrich, RN, MS, CCRN

Airlift Northwest, 6311 49th Avenue SW, Seattle, WA 98136, USA

Maintenance of adequate tissue perfusion is a major goal in the management of the critically ill. Traditionally, vital signs, such as pulse, blood pressure, mentation, and urine output, have been used as therapeutic end points for correction of imbalances in systemic oxygenation. These parameters are poor indicators of ongoing tissue hypoxia [1]. Early correction of imbalances between oxygen delivery and consumption to relieve tissue hypoxia decreases morbidity and mortality in the critically ill [2,3].

Continuous monitoring and evaluation of tissue oxygenation at the bedside is accomplished by using a fiberoptic, pulmonary artery catheter to measure mixed venous oxygen saturation (SvO_2). Clinically, SvO_2 is used to guide resuscitation, because it indicates the presence of ongoing global tissue hypoxia in the critically ill [4]; however, it always may not be feasible to place a pulmonary artery catheter to measure continuous SvO_2 early in resuscitation or outside of the ICU. Recently, a technology that uses a modified central venous catheter with fiberoptic technology was introduced into clinical practice. Placement of a central line is considered standard of care for most critical care patients [5]. Central venous catheterization has less associated risks and is easier to perform than is placement of a pulmonary artery catheter [5]. Central venous oxygen saturation ($ScvO_2$) monitoring is now being used before, or as an alternative to, placement of a fiberoptic pulmonary artery catheter in many settings, including the Emergency Department (ED). This new technology allows for measurement of $ScvO_2$ in the superior vena cava (SVC), which has been shown to trend with SvO_2. Continuous monitoring of SvO_2 and $ScvO_2$ has proven to be beneficial in the early identification and treatment of patients who have global tissue hypoxia, even when vital signs seem to be normal [1,6,7].

Using continuous $ScvO_2$ monitoring to evaluate tissue oxygenation at the bedside enables the clinician to detect early alterations in oxygen balance. This allows for aggressive implementation of therapeutic interventions that are aimed at restoring oxygen balance.

Overview

To appreciate the clinical significance of $ScvO_2$, it is necessary to have a fundamental understanding of the principles of oxygen delivery and consumption. Oxygen delivery is the amount of oxygen that is delivered to the tissues per minute. It is determined by cardiac output (CO), hemoglobin (Hb), and arterial oxygen saturation (SaO_2).

Oxygen consumption is the amount of oxygen that is used by the tissues per minute. Oxygen consumption varies between different tissues. Highly metabolic tissues (heart) consume more oxygen, whereas less metabolic tissues (skin) consume less oxygen. Normally, the tissues use only 25% of the delivered oxygen. In a stress state, tissue metabolism is increased, and less oxygen returns to the heart.

Homeostasis within the body is maintained by balancing oxygen delivery and oxygen consumption. When oxygen supply (delivery) decreases or oxygen demand (consumption) increases, this delicate balance is threatened. When an imbalance occurs, compensatory mechanisms are activated to ensure

The author is a senior education consultant for Edwards Lifesciences, Irvine, California.

E-mail address: goodrichc@aol.com

adequate oxygen availability to meet the metabolic demands of the tissues. Compensatory mechanisms that are available immediately include increased CO and increased oxygen extraction. Compromised cardiac function may limit the body's ability to maximize CO as a mechanism to meet increasing metabolic needs. When this occurs, tissue oxygen extraction increases and less oxygen returns to the lungs to be reoxygenated. When oxygen demands exceed supply or when oxygen delivery is compromised, a decrease in SvO_2 is seen. If compensatory mechanisms fail to restore the balance between oxygen supply and demand, anaerobic metabolism, lactic acidosis, and global tissue hypoxia result [8]. Therefore, SvO_2 may serve as a global indicator of the balance between oxygen delivery and oxygen demand.

Definitions of mixed and central venous oxygen saturation

SvO_2 is measured using a fiberoptic, pulmonary artery catheter. It reflects the overall, oxygen saturation of blood returning from the inferior vena cava (IVC; lower body), superior vena cava (upper body), and the coronary sinus (heart). Variations in regional blood flow from the SVC, IVC, and coronary sinus affect the absolute values of $ScvO_2$ and SvO_2 [9].

Placing a fiberoptic, central venous catheter into the SVC allows for measurement of $ScvO_2$, which reflects blood returning from the upper body, and indicates oxygen balance in the cranial portion of the body, including the brain [9].

Physiologic relationship between mixed venous and superior vena cava oxygen saturation

Several clinical studies have examined the relationship between SvO_2 and $ScvO_2$ [5,10–13]. This relationship varies, depending upon the health or disease state of the individual. The difference between SvO_2 and $ScvO_2$ is the result of distribution of CO within the body. SvO_2 that is measured using a pulmonary artery catheter reflects blood returning from the upper body, lower body, and the heart. It is a measure of total body oxygen saturation. $ScvO_2$ reflects blood returning from the upper body including the brain.

In healthy individuals, SvO_2 normally is higher than $ScvO_2$ [5]. This occurs because the kidneys receive a higher proportion of CO, but use less oxygen [14]. More oxygen returns from the lower body, and oxygen saturation is increased in the IVC [10,11].

In pathologic states, such as severe sepsis [5,12,13], circulatory shock [10], cardiac shock [11], heart failure [11], and head injury [5], this relationship

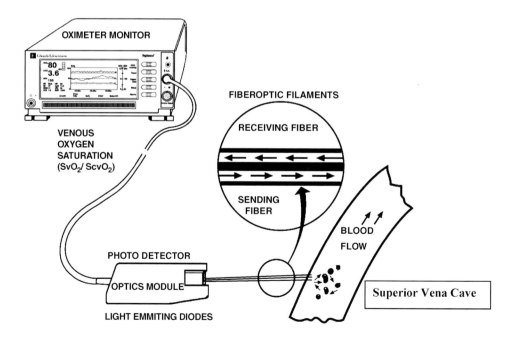

Fig. 1. Overview of reflection spectrophotometry. (Courtesy of Edwards Lifesciences, Irvine, CA; with permission.)

changes and ScvO$_2$ is generally higher than SvO$_2$. When shock occurs, blood flow to the vital organs, including the brain and heart, is maintained. At the same time, there is decreased blood flow to the kidneys and splanchnic circulations. This causes a decrease in the oxygen saturation of blood that is returning from the lower body (IVC), and results in ScvO$_2$ being greater than SvO$_2$ [7,11,15]. These studies suggest that a low ScvO$_2$ indicates an even lower SvO$_2$.

Although ScvO$_2$ and SvO$_2$ values do not correlate absolutely, they have been shown to trend with one another over a variety of changing clinical conditions [5]. Using continuous ScvO$_2$ monitoring as a surrogate for SvO$_2$ enhances decision making in nontraditional settings, such as the ED or stepdown unit.

Measurement

Equipment that is needed to measure continuous ScvO$_2$ includes a fiberoptic, central venous catheter; optic module cable; and a specialized computer (Fig. 1). A modified, triple-lumen, central venous catheter is placed into the SVC. This catheter also allows for fluid administration and measurement of central venous pressure (CVP). Selected wavelengths of light are transmitted down one fiberoptic filament in the catheter to the blood flowing past the catheter tip in the SVC. A second fiberoptic filament transmits the reflected light back to a photodetector that is located in the optic module cable. The reflected light is analyzed to determine ScvO$_2$, because oxyhemoglobin and hemoglobin absorb light at different wavelengths. This results in the display of a continuous, real-time ScvO$_2$ reading on the monitor screen.

Interpretation of continuous central venous oxygen saturation

Normal and abnormalities in continuous central venous oxygen saturation

A target ScvO$_2$ value of 70% or greater is used to guide therapy in the critically ill [5,13]. It is common for individuals who have cardiopulmonary compromise to have alterations in ScvO$_2$. Changes in ScvO$_2$ indicate an imbalance between oxygen delivery and consumption. When this occurs, an immediate evaluation of the components of oxygen delivery (CO, SaO$_2$, Hb) and oxygen consumption is indicated.

Identification of the factors that precipitated the imbalance allow for timely institution of appropriate therapeutic interventions. Re-evaluation of ScvO$_2$ indicates whether the identified interventions have restored oxygen balance.

A decrease in ScvO$_2$ is caused by a decrease in oxygen delivery or an increase in oxygen consumption. Many clinical conditions can precipitate these imbalances (Box 1). An increase in ScvO$_2$ results when there is an increase in oxygen delivery or a decrease in oxygen consumption.

Clinical application

Continuous ScvO$_2$ has been used in a variety of settings for the early management of patients who have severe sepsis and septic shock [13], cardiac

---

Box 1. Causes of altered central and mixed venous oxygen saturation

High central and mixed venous oxygen saturation

Increased oxygen delivery
↑ Cardiac output
↑ Hemoglobin level
↑ Arterial oxygen saturation

Decreased oxygen consumption
Pharmacologic paralysis
Hypothermia,
Anesthesia
Late sepsis

Low central and mixed venous oxygen saturation

Decreased oxygen delivery
↓ Cardiac output
↓ Hemoglobin level
↓ Arterial oxygen saturation

Increased oxygen consumption
Shivering
Fever
Pain
Shivering
Seizures
Increased work of breathing
Agitation

arrest [16–18], acutely decompensated congestive heart failure (CHF) [19], or traumatic and hemorrhagic shock; [7,20]; following resuscitation after cardiac arrest [8], and in high-risk surgical patients [21,22].

Severe sepsis and septic shock

Global tissue hypoxia has been described well in the literature; it develops before severe sepsis, septic shock, multiorgan failure, and death [23]. Traditional measurements of hemodynamic pressures and vital signs, such as blood pressure and heart rate, have been found to be poor indicators of ongoing global tissue hypoxia [1].

Recently, continuous $ScvO_2$ monitoring was studied as a resuscitation end point in the management of severe sepsis and septic shock [13]. Rivers and colleagues [13] evaluated the use of early goal-directed therapy (EGDT) as a systematic approach to the management of septic patients (Fig. 2). One of the primary goals of EGDT is prompt restoration of oxygen balance. In this study, an EGDT protocol was implemented on admission to the ED, before transfer to the ICU. Patients who had severe sepsis or septic shock who presented to the ED were randomized to

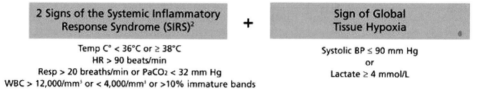
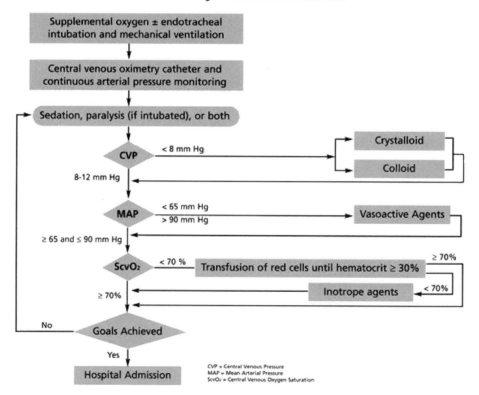

Fig. 2. Early goal-directed therapy. (Courtesy of Edwards Lifesciences, Irvine, CA; with permission.)

receive 6 hours EGDT or 6 hours of standard sepsis care. A total of 263 patients was enrolled in the study; 130 received EGDT and 133 received standard treatment. The major therapeutic targets were the same for both groups. These included achieving a CVP of 8 to 12 mm Hg and a mean arterial pressure (MAP) of greater than 65 mm Hg. Additionally, those who received EGDT also were resuscitated to a continuous $ScvO_2$ value of 70% or greater.

The in-hospital mortality for patients who received standard treatment was 46.5%, but was 30.5% in the group that received EGDT ($P = .009$). During the first 72 hours, the group that received EGDT had lower lactate levels and base deficits, higher mean $ScvO_2$ values, and lower Acute Physiology and Chronic Health Evaluation II scores; these indicated less organ dysfunction. Overall study results showed that in-hospital mortality was reduced by 16% and length of stay was decreased by approximately 3.8 days in patients who received EGDT.

Acutely decompensated congestive heart failure

An acute deterioration in myocardial function can lead to cardiogenic shock, which results in global tissue hypoxia [19]. Ander and colleagues [19] studied the use of continuous $ScvO_2$ and lactic acid levels and as a way of stratifying and managing 27 patients who were admitted to the ED with acutely decompensated, end-stage, chronic CHF (ejection fraction <30%). They used a prospective, non-outcome, convenience sampling design to study patients who were admitted to an urban tertiary care hospital. This group was subdivided into patients who had normal (≤ 2 mM/L; n = 5) or high lactic acid (>2 mM/L; n = 22) levels. Seventeen stable patients who presented to the cardiology clinic were used as matched controls. Patients were managed using a standardized protocol that included evaluation of lactic acid levels and continuous $ScvO_2$ monitoring. Therapeutic interventions that were guided by continuous $ScvO_2$ monitoring resulted in significantly decreased lactic acid levels, and which indicated resolving global tissue hypoxia.

These investigators concluded that the use of continuous $ScvO_2$ monitoring and lactic acid levels was superior to the use of vital signs in identifying and managing patients who had occult cardiogenic shock. Early identification of occult cardiogenic shock allowed for aggressive management strategies that were aimed at resolution of global tissue hypoxia in the ED. These investigators also noted the need to investigate the impact of monitoring continuous $ScvO_2$ and lactic acid levels on overall health care costs, morbidity, and mortality.

Cardiac arrest

A major goal during cardiopulmonary resuscitation (CPR) is to re-establish spontaneous circulation, and thereby, provide oxygen delivery to vital organs. Commonly, physical examination findings, cardiac rhythm analysis, and vital signs are used to guide the resuscitation of victims of cardiac arrest.

Several studies have evaluated the usefulness of continuous $ScvO_2$ monitoring and central venous oxygen tension ($PcvO_2$) measurements as diagnostic and treatment guides during cardiac arrest [16,24]. Rivers and colleagues [24] described the changes that occurred in continuous $ScvO_2$ during CPR and immediately after return of spontaneous circulation (ROSC). The study included 100 patients who presented to the ED with normothermic, nontraumatic cardiac arrest. Sixty-eight episodes of cardiac arrest were studied. Patients who had ROSC had statistically higher values of $ScvO_2$, $PcvO_2$, and pH. ROSC was observed in all patients who attained $ScvO_2$ values of greater than 72%, ROSC did not occur in any patient who had a $ScvO_2$ value of less than 30%, and only 1 patient attained ROSC without attaining an $ScvO_2$ of 40%. These investigators concluded that continuous $ScvO_2$ monitoring is a valuable tool to guide treatment during resuscitation, and is predictive of ROSC in victims of cardiac arrest.

Snyder and colleagues [16] investigated the use of $PcvO_2$ as a predictor of outcome during CPR. Over a 9-month period, 43 patients who required intubation and CPR were studied in a community teaching hospital. Only 33% of the patients survived for at least 24 hours after resuscitation. At 10 minutes, all survivors had a $PcvO_2$ value of at least 41 mm Hg. These investigators concluded that $PcvO_2$ seems to be a valuable predictor of poor outcome in hospitalized victims of cardiac arrest.

Postresuscitation after cardiac arrest

Continued hemodynamic instability frequently is a cause of rearrest after resuscitation of victims of cardiac arrest. $ScvO_2$ monitoring is useful in detecting ongoing oxygen imbalances that might not have resolved fully during resuscitation. Rivers and colleagues [8] stated that in the postresuscitation period, $ScvO_2$ values of greater than 60% to 70% indicate hemodynamic stability, but a decrease in $ScvO_2$ to less than 40% to 50% indicates that the patient is at risk for rearrest.

Trauma and hemorrhagic shock

Immediate assessment and aggressive management strategies are the cornerstones of treatment for patients who have sustained trauma. Frequently, evaluation and treatment are guided by the use of vital signs, such as pulse and blood pressure. Studies of patients who have sustained trauma showed that vital signs are unreliable resuscitation end points [7,20].

Rady and colleagues [25] observed that 50% of patients who were in shock and who were stabilized using vital signs, such as pulse and blood pressure, still had a low $ScvO_2$ value. These investigators found that patients who had $ScvO_2$ values of less than 65% had increased lactate levels and prolonged cardiac dysfunction, which indicated the need for further resuscitation.

Another study by Scalea and colleagues [7] investigated the usefulness of central venous oxygen saturation (CVO_2) as a tool to detect blood loss in patients who had sustained trauma patients and were admitted to the ED. These authors studied 26 patients who were admitted to the ED with a trauma mechanism that was suggestive of blood loss. All of the patients were assessed as being stable after the initial evaluation. Most patients (21 of 26) had penetrating injuries. Blood pressure, pulse, pulse pressure, CVP, urine output, and CVO_2 were evaluated in each patient. Thirty-nine percent of the patients had a CVO_2 of less than 65%; all required blood transfusions. These patients also had larger amounts of estimated blood loss and more severe injuries. The investigators concluded that CVO_2 is a more reliable indicator of blood loss in patients who have sustained trauma. In addition, CVO_2 can assist in the early identification of patients who will require blood transfusions.

High-risk surgical patients

Several researchers have begun to evaluate the clinical usefulness of continuous $ScvO_2$ monitoring in high-risk surgery patients [21,22]. Pearse and colleagues [21] investigated the use of continuous $ScvO_2$ monitoring as a predictor of mortality in 12 high-risk patients who underwent surgery. $ScvO_2$ values were recorded for the first 8 hours postoperatively, and were used as a guide for resuscitation. The authors found that postoperative values for $ScvO_2$ of less than 65% were predictive of increased mortality in this population.

In another study, Pearse and colleagues [22] studied the use of continuous $ScvO_2$ monitoring in 79 high-risk patients who underwent surgery and who were evaluated postoperatively for the first 8 hours. These patients were followed for 28 days. Patients were divided into groups that had low ($<65\%$ for at least 2 consecutive hours) and high ($>65\%$) levels of $ScvO_2$. The investigators found that low levels of $ScvO_2$ were associated with a higher prevalence of cardiac complications and sepsis, longer hospital length of stays, and a trend toward higher mortality. They concluded that in this population, a low level of $ScvO_2$ was predictive of a higher risk for postoperative complications, and it was more predictive of hypovolemia than are traditional measures, such as blood pressure, pulse, and serum lactate level.

Summary

Restoration of oxygen balance is a major goal in the treatment of the critically ill [13,26]. Traditionally, this has been accomplished by placing a pulmonary artery catheter in the ICU to monitor tissue oxygenation at the bedside. Unfortunately, placement of pulmonary artery catheters is not always possible in areas outside of the ICU environment. Introduction of continuous $ScvO_2$ monitoring that uses a modified, central venous catheter makes it possible to evaluate ongoing tissue oxygenation in nontraditional settings. Although SvO_2 and $ScvO_2$ values do not correlate absolutely, they do trend with one another. Continuous $ScvO_2$ monitoring is becoming a valuable tool for evaluation during resuscitation in the ED where placement of a central venous catheter is routinely used to manage patients.

Many studies showed that vital signs and other hemodynamic parameters, such as heart pressures, are inadequate indicators of existing tissue oxygenation imbalances [7,13,20]. $ScvO_2$ provides the clinician with a continuous, real-time parameter that allows for evaluation of tissue oxygenation at the bedside. Similar to continuous SvO_2, $ScvO_2$ monitoring allows for immediate feedback that is related to the effectiveness of therapeutic interventions. It also provides early warning and surveillance for changes in a patient's ability to provide adequate oxygen supply to meet metabolic demands.

References

[1] Rady MY, Rivers EP, Norwalk RM. Resuscitation of the critically ill in the ED: response of blood pressure, heart rate, shock index, central venous oxygen saturation, and lactate. Am J Emerg Med 1996;14:218–25.

[2] Boyd O, Grounds RM, Bennett D. A randomized clinical trial of the effect of deliberate peri-operative increase of oxygen delivery on mortality in high-risk surgical patients. JAMA 1993;270:2699–707.

[3] Tuchschmidt J, Fried J, Astiz M, et al. Elevation of cardiac output and oxygen delivery improves outcome in septic shock. Chest 1992;102:216–20.

[4] Dickens JJ. Central venous oxygenation saturation monitoring: a role for critical care? Curr Anaesth Crit Care 2004;15:378–82.

[5] Reinhart K, Huhn HJ, Hartog C, et al. Continuous central venous and pulmonary artery oxygen saturation monitoring in the critically ill. Intensive Care Med 2004;30:1572–8.

[6] Rady MY, Rivers EP, Martin GB, et al. Continuous central venous oximetry and shock index in the emergency department. Am J Emerg Med 1992;10:538–41.

[7] Scalea TM, Hartnett RW, Duncan AO, et al. Central venous oxygen saturation: a useful tool in trauma patients. J Trauma 1990;30:1539–43.

[8] Rivers EP, Ander DS, Powell D. Central venous oxygen saturation monitoring in the critically ill patient. Curr Opin Crit Care 2001;7(3):204–11.

[9] Turnaoglu S, Tugrul M, Camci E, et al. Clinical applicability of the substitution of mixed venous oxygen saturation with central venous oxygen saturation. J Cardiothorac Vasc Anesth 2001;15(5):574–9.

[10] Lee J, Wright F, Barber R, et al. Central venous oxygen saturation in shock: a study in man. Anesthesiology 1972;36:472–8.

[11] Scheinman MM, Brown MA, Rapaort E. Critical assessment of use of central venous oxygen saturation as a mirror of mixed venous oxygen saturation in severely ill cardiac patients. Circulation 1969;40:165–70.

[12] Dahn MS, Lange MP, Jacobs LA. Central mixed and splanchnic venous oxygen saturation monitoring. Intensive Care Med 1988;14:373–8.

[13] Rivers EP, Nguyen B, Havstad S, et al. Early goal directed therapy in the treatment of severe sepsis and septic shock. N Engl J Med 2001;345(19):1368–77.

[14] Cargill W, Hickman J. The oxygen consumption of the normal and disease human kidney. J Clin Invest 1949;28:526–9.

[15] Edwards JD, Mayall RM. Importance of the sampling site for measurement of mixed venous oxygen saturation in shock. Crit Care Med 1998;26:1356–60.

[16] Snyder AB, Salloum LJ, Barone JE, et al. Predicting short-term outcome of cardiopulmonary resuscitation using central venous oxygen tension measurements. Crit Care Med 1991;19:111–3.

[17] Nakazawa K, Hikawa Y, Saitoh Y, et al. Usefulness of central venous oxygen saturation monitoring during cardiopulmonary resuscitation: a comparative case study with end-tidal carbon dioxide monitoring. Intensive Care Med 1994;20:450–1.

[18] Paradis NA, Martin GB, Goetting MG, et al. Aortic pressure during human cardiac arrest: identification of pseudo-electromechanical dissociation. Chest 1992;101:123–8.

[19] Anders DS, Jaggi M, Rivers E, et al. Undetected cardiogenic shock in patients with congestive heart failure presenting to the emergency department. Am J Cardiol 1998;82:888–991.

[20] Wo CC, Shoemaker WC, Appel PL, et al. Unreliability of blood pressure and heart rate to evaluate cardiac output in emergency resuscitation and critical illness. Crit Care Med 1993;21:218–23.

[21] Pearse R, Dawson D, Rhodes A, et al. Low central venous saturation predicts post-operative mortality. Presented at the 16th Annual Cardiac Surgery Congress. Amsterdam, 2003.

[22] Pearse R, Dawson D, Fawcett J, et al. The relationship between central venous saturation and outcome following high-risk surgery [abstract]. Crit Care 2004;8(Suppl 1):P51.

[23] Beal AL, Cerra FB. Multiple organ failure syndrome in the 1990's: systemic inflammatory response and organ dysfunction. JAMA 1994;271:226–33.

[24] Rivers EP, Martin GB, Smithline H, et al. The clinical implications of continuous central venous oxygen saturation during human CPR. Ann Emerg Med 1992;21(9):1094–101.

[25] Rady MY, Rivers EP, Martin GB, et al. Continuous central venous oximetry and shock index in the emergency department: use in the evaluation of clinical shock. Am J Emerg Med 1992;10:538–41.

[26] Nelson LD. Continuous venous oximetry in surgical patients. Ann Surg 1986;203(3):329–33.

ELSEVIER
SAUNDERS

Crit Care Nurs Clin N Am 18 (2006) 211 – 215

CRITICAL CARE
NURSING CLINICS
OF NORTH AMERICA

Transcutaneous Carbon Dioxide Monitoring

Kathleen M. Hill, MSN, RN, CCNS[a,*], Deborah G. Klein, MSN, RN, CCRN, CS[b,c]

[a]Cardiothoracic Intensive Care Units, Cleveland Clinic, 9500 Euclid Avenue, P-32, Cleveland, OH 44195, USA
[b]Cardiac Intensive Care Unit and Heart Failure Special Care Unit, Cleveland Clinic, 9500 Euclid Avenue, P-32, Cleveland, OH 44195, USA
[c]Frances Payne Bolton School of Nursing, Case Western Reserve University, Cleveland, OH USA

For the last 15 years, monitoring of oxygen saturation levels has enabled practitioners to assess changes in oxygenation, perfusion, and ventilation. Pulse oximetry has provided a method to assess oxygenation parameters without an arterial blood gas. Technologies now exist, however, that can detect rising and falling carbon dioxide (CO_2) levels through noninvasive mechanisms. CO_2, the by-product of energy production levels, can be measured from a variety of sources including the bronchus (end-tidal CO_2 device), under the tongue (sublingual probe), and through the skin (transcutaneous probe) to provide the critical care practitioner with additional information about ventilation, perfusion, and metabolism. Noninvasive measures of CO_2 production can validate or negate the need for more costly and higher risk monitoring technology such as the pulmonary artery catheter [1,2]. Rapid assessment of the patient who has signs of depressed ventilatory effort or sepsis can aid in treatment decisions such as whether further monitoring is needed in an ICU setting.

This article describes the rationale for using CO_2 levels obtained through transcutaneous CO_2 ($TctCO_2$) monitoring as a method to evaluate symptoms of hypoventilation and depressed perfusion. The benefits, indications, and a description of this continuous, noninvasive technology are presented.

Pathophysiology

The lungs support the functions of ventilation and respiration. Ventilation involves the movement of a gas (oxygen) into the alveolus, followed by removal of a gas (CO_2) from an adjacent capillary. CO_2 is the by-product of metabolic activity in the cell. It is transported from the cells, dissolved in plasma or bound to plasma proteins and hemoglobin, and excreted through the lungs. The lungs serve as a conduit for passive removal of CO_2 from the cell as it moves across the capillary of the lungs, through the alveolar membrane, and exits the bronchial tree into the atmosphere. Its excretion depends on the ability to cross the capillary and be pulled into the alveolus for eventual excretion through the mechanism of exhalation. The exchange of CO_2 and oxygen at the tissue level through capillary interface supports cellular energy metabolism. As oxygen is consumed by the cell, CO_2 is produced as a by-product of aerobic metabolism. Decreased perfusion or flow through the capillary results in decreased clearance of CO_2 and an accumulation of CO_2 in the capillary. Box 1 lists conditions that increase and decrease CO_2 production [3]. The CO_2 that remains in the capillary can be measured through a transcutaneous sensor [4,5].

History

Transcutaneous monitoring of CO_2 has been used for more than 30 years in neonates and infants [4]. A calibrated probe is placed on a well-perfused area of

* Corresponding author.
E-mail address: hillk4@ccf.org (K.M. Hill).

Box 1. Conditions that increase and decrease carbon dioxide production

Increased carbon dioxide production

   Activity
   Hyperthyroidism
   Trauma
   Burns
   High carbohydrate intake
   Sepsis
   Hyperthermia

Decreased carbon dioxide production

   Sedation
   Paralysis
   Hypothyroidism
   Hypothermia

the trunk or thigh and heated to a temperature between 42°C and 44°C to increase perfusion to the area. The electrode measures the amount of CO_2 diffused through the skin and displays a number on a monitor. This technique decreases the need for frequent arterial blood gas sampling. Technical concerns related to calibration of the equipment and the need to rotate sensor sites to avoid thermal injury to the skin have slowed its introduction in the adult population [5].

In the adult population, trends toward noninvasive monitoring of hemodynamic function and perfusion are not new, as evidenced by the emergence of thoracic impedance cardiac output devices, pulse contour cardiac output, and pulse oximetry. Transcutaneous monitoring of CO_2 follows this trend toward noninvasive monitoring by limiting the need for arterial blood gas analysis.

Research

Janssens and colleagues [1], in a Swiss study of 26 healthy volunteers, found excellent correlation between $TctCO_2$ measurements and arterial measurement of CO_2. Hourly sampling was performed over a 4-hour period in 4 of the subjects. Six subjects received noninvasive positive-pressure ventilation while arterial and $TctCO_2$ levels were measured. Transcutaneous and arterial levels of CO_2 were comparable following this change in ventilatory

mode. Although there was excellent agreement in the data, study limitations included a small sample size and stable subjects.

Rosner and colleagues' [6] French study of 10 adult patients concluded that the $TctCO_2$ measurement provided a reliable estimate of the arterial blood gas level of CO_2. This 1999 study also compared arterial blood gas measurement of CO_2 with transcutaneous sources. Subjects were hospitalized adults who had severe chronic respiratory failure requiring nocturnal ventilatory support. Measurement of transcutaneous and arterial blood gases were collected six times at 1-hour intervals. The results did not vary over time, provided that an initial arterial blood gas sample was obtained for calibration with the transcutaneous value. The study was small in size and enrolled only hemodynamically stable adults.

High $TctCO_2$ values correlated well with mortality in 48 trauma patients, as reported by Tatevossian and coworkers [7] in 2000. This descriptive study of severely injured patients presenting to a level I trauma center in Los Angeles, California, sought to compare patterns of tissue perfusion by measuring $TctCO_2$ over time. Immediately after hospital admission, the $TctCO_2$ was used as an early sign of poor tissue perfusion, producing a time pattern that could be related to survivors and nonsurvivors. Nonsurvivors demonstrated higher $TctCO_2$ levels early in the course of therapy—within the first hour of admission. Elevated $TctCO_2$ levels were associated with a 100% mortality rate when those levels were sustained for more than 30 minutes. The investigators concluded that $TctCO_2$ and oxygen monitoring might act as an early indicator of tissue hypoxia, hypovolemia, and hemodynamic shock in severely ill patients during the early emergency department period. The critically ill subjects and larger sample size made this study result more applicable to the hospitalized population.

Lagerkvist and colleagues [8] demonstrated in 2003 that $TctCO_2$ monitoring results could be reliably produced over time. This Swedish study of 41 healthy children and adolescents sought to establish the degree of variation in transcutaneous oxygen tension, CO_2 tension, and oxygen saturation values between and within individual subjects. Results indicated that the transcutaneous values are reliable estimates of blood gas tension. The investigators cautioned that results from the healthy subjects could not automatically be translated to the ill.

Griffin and colleagues [9] in 2003 studied 30 adults undergoing gastric bypass surgery. In several obese patients (body mass index >40) undergoing general anesthesia, the researchers found that $TctCO_2$ was comparable to the arterial CO_2 levels.

End-tidal CO$_2$ measurements were not as close as TctCO$_2$ to the arterial blood gas value.

Tobias [10] published similar results in 2003 after evaluating the accuracy of TctCO$_2$ versus end-tidal CO$_2$ devices during one-lung ventilation anesthesia in 15 patients undergoing thoracic surgical procedures. The TctCO$_2$ and end-tidal CO$_2$ devices were used simultaneously in each study subject while comparing arterial CO$_2$ tension. The TctCO$_2$ method displayed greater accuracy with the arterial source than the end-tidal CO$_2$ device. The studies undertaken by Griffin and colleagues [9] and Tobias [10] were limited in size but their subjects reflected patients commonly found in the hospital environment.

Hasibeder and coworkers [2] demonstrated a linear relationship between TctCO$_2$ levels and partial pressure of CO$_2$ in a 1991 publication. The study, set among 24 critically ill adults, could not link TctCO$_2$ with the hemodynamic data of cardiac index and mean arterial pressure. Each participant was entered into the study because he or she was being monitored with a pulmonary artery catheter. The reasons for admission to the ICU were related to an assortment of common medical and surgical diagnoses. As in other studies, arterial and TctCO$_2$ levels were obtained simultaneously, compared, and found to have a linear correlation. The investigators suggested that alterations in TctCO$_2$, without changes in arterial CO$_2$, reflect changes in blood flow. In low-flow states, lactic acid accumulates in the skin and is buffered, producing more CO$_2$ that can be reflected in the TctCO$_2$ level. These low-flow states also slow the exit of CO$_2$, contributing to more skin accumulation of CO$_2$. The investigators concluded that TctCO$_2$ could assist in identifying early changes in perfusion caused by vasoconstriction.

Transcutaneous carbon dioxide measurement

CO$_2$ production and accumulation can be measured invasively through arterial blood gas analysis and noninvasively through end-tidal measurement, sublingually, and by the transcutaneous route.

Arterial blood gas sampling of CO$_2$ levels remains the "gold standard" for estimating the adequacy of ventilatory support. End-tidal CO$_2$ measurement can be a reflection of the adequacy of blood flow and delivery of CO$_2$ to the alveolus and the clearance of CO$_2$ from the alveolus [11]. Sublingual monitoring of CO$_2$ has been used in conditions in which the gastrointestinal system has been deprived of adequate perfusion, such as in early stages of shock. It is an intermittent measurement, not a continuous one,

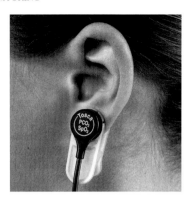

Fig. 1. Placement of earlobe sensor for TctCO$_2$ monitoring. (Courtesy of Radiometer America, Westlake, OH; with permission.)

requiring the nurse to use a probe to acquire each data point [11].

Transcutaneous measurement of CO$_2$ uses a calibrated probe placed on the trunk, thigh, abdomen, or earlobe (Fig. 1). Calibration [1,8] is done by exposing the probe to a known concentration of CO$_2$ (5%, 10%, or room air). The probe is continuously heated to a temperature between 42°C and 44°C. Heating the probe increases perfusion to the area by promoting maximal vasodilatation and the loss of autoregulation [2]. At these high local temperatures, the skin's vessels do not dilate or constrict but serve as passive conduits for blood flow. Therefore, the hyperemia induced by application of the skin electrode is necessary to measure TctCO$_2$. Blood flow is dependent on regional skin perfusion, which is determined by systemic perfusion pressure.

The monitoring device provides a digital reading of the partial pressure of CO$_2$ and oxygen saturation (SpO$_2$) levels, pulse rate, and a continuous graphic reading of the pulse waveform (Fig. 2). Physiologic conditions that benefit from this type of monitoring include respiratory insufficiency and acute tissue perfusion deficits such sepsis or local occlusion [12]. Other applications include validation of the need for additional invasive measures such as pulmonary artery catheterization and validation of those patients requiring further monitoring in an ICU but awaiting transfer [12].

Advantages and limitations

Transcutaneous monitoring of CO$_2$ levels reflects arterial CO$_2$ levels [4,5,8–10]. The advantage of continuous measurement in a noninvasive, blood-sparing monitor makes this a very attractive method

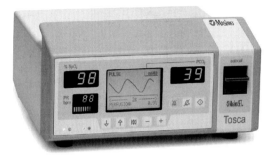

Fig. 2. TOSCA 500 noninvasive device for monitoring TctCO$_2$, SpO$_2$, and pulse rate through a single sensor. (Courtesy of Radiometer America, Westlake, OH; with permission.)

of data acquisition. TctCO$_2$ monitoring can provide an early warning of circulatory collapse and shock by identifying situations of increased production of CO$_2$ in the periphery. The TctCO$_2$ method can provide a continuous evaluation of CO$_2$ production and clearance from peripheral tissues. TctCO$_2$ monitoring assesses the metabolic activity, systemic circulation, and local perfusion of tissues.

Limitations associated with the technique include the consideration that TctCO$_2$ monitoring is new compared with the universal use of arterial blood gas and end-tidal CO$_2$ measurements. The monitoring technology has not been widely used in the United States, although numerous studies in the European adult population have been published [1,2,6,8]. In the United States, this technology has been studied and applied primarily in the neonatal population, which makes it prudent to view it with some reservation until it can prove its utility over time and in large adult populations. Monitoring systems available for adult use have been developed and marketed by companies such as Linde Medical Sensors and Masimo Corporation [13,14]. The newer-generation devices allow for faster calibration (2 minutes) than the original equipment [13,14]. As a rule of safety, investigators have recommended moving the skin sensor every 4 hours to avoid skin burn [1]. This precaution may be seen as a limitation because it adds an extra nursing intervention to the monitoring process. The detection of CO$_2$ levels through the skin is dependent on flow/perfusion to the region where the sensor is applied and may not be indicative of tissue perfusion within the entire body [6]. The learning curve should also be considered when introducing a new technology and a different approach in interpreting physiologic data. Although nurses and other health care practitioners may be intimately familiar with the interaction between the principles of blood flow/perfusion, ventilation, and

Box 2. Advantages and limitations of the transcutaneous method of carbon dioxide monitoring

Advantages

Noninvasive
No introduction of pathogens
Blood-sparing
Timesaving, with minimal set-up and calibration [13,14]
Instant readings
Decreased risk of operator error
No apparent difference with increased body mass index [15]
Early recognition of poor tissue perfusion from low flow states
Early recognition of airway occlusion as cause of rising CO$_2$ levels
May provide early warning of low fluid volume or circulatory collapse [7]
May provide early warning of alveolar hypoventilation in patients being weaned from mechanical ventilation
May assist in evaluation of patients on t-piece trials or other weaning protocols
Assists in distinguishing respiratory depression/hypoventilation as cause of change in LOC
Continuous data display [13,14]
Not influenced by lung disease or other ventilation-perfusion disorders
Cost savings: reduces need for frequent arterial blood gases
Less painful due to decrease in number of arterial sticks for blood gas analysis
Assists in decisions to intubate and initiate mechanical ventilation
Assists in determining optimal ventilator settings

Limitations

No history: has time proved its value?
May limit reliability in decreased cardiac output, vasoconstriction, or hypothermia, especially if cardiac index is less than 1.5 L/min/cm^2 [16]
Skin site change every 4 hours to avoid burning at sensor site [1]

Tension of CO_2 at one skin segment may not be reflective of all tissues [7]

Calibration required every 4 to 6 hours; accuracy directly linked to skin perfusion [17]

cellular metabolism, the introduction of new linkages and methods of interpreting data may take some time to incorporate into practice. Box 2 summarizes the advantages and limitations of this technology [1,7,13–17].

Summary

TctCO$_2$ measurement can be helpful in evaluating ventilation and perfusion. The pulmonary contribution to hemodynamic function can be articulated through an assessment of oxygenation and ventilation. The SpO$_2$ device provides rapid, reliable data, reflective of the oxygenation function of the lungs. The by-product of ventilation, CO_2, can now be quantified, tracked real-time, and trended using the TctCO$_2$ probe and monitor. Thus, TctCO$_2$ measurements are complementary to SpO$_2$ data.

The benefit of TctCO$_2$ monitoring may be its ability to alert the practitioner early in the course of decreased circulatory flow or decreased ventilatory effort. Both events—poor flow and poor gas exchange—create a condition in which there is accumulation of CO_2 on the skin. This noninvasive technology can offer alternatives to more complex, costly, and resource-intensive data acquisition such as arterial blood gases, arterial catheters, pulmonary artery catheters, and other tools that are used to determine markers of tissue perfusion.

References

[1] Janssens JP, Haworth-Frey C, Chevrolet JC, et al. Transcutaneous Pco2 to monitor noninvasive mechanical ventilation in adults. Chest 1998;113:768–73.

[2] Hasibeder W, Haisjack M, Sparr H, et al. Factors influencing transcutaneous oxygen and carbon dioxide measurements in adult intensive care patients. Intensive Care Med 1991;17:272–5.

[3] Hess D, Tobin MJ. Capnometry. In: Tobin MJ, editor. Principles and practice of intensive care monitoring. New York: McGraw-Hill; 1998. p. 377–93.

[4] Lubbers D. Theoretical basis of the transcutaneous blood gas measurements. Crit Care Med 1981;9(10): 721–33.

[5] Thomas P. What's the latest on carbon dioxide monitoring? Neonatal Netw 2004;23(4):70–2.

[6] Rosner V, Hannart B, Cabot F, et al. Validity of transcutaneous oxygen/carbon dioxide pressure measurement in the monitoring of mechanical ventilation in stable chronic respiratory failure. Eur Respir J 1999; 13:1044–7.

[7] Tatevossian R, Wo C, Velmahos G, et al. Transcutaneous oxygen and CO_2 as early warning of tissue hypoxia and hemodynamic shock in critically ill emergency patients. Crit Care Med 2000;28(7): 2248–53.

[8] Lagerkvist AL, Sten G, Redfors S, et al. Repeated blood gas monitoring in healthy children and adolescents by the transcutaneous route. Pediatr Pulmonol 2003;35:274–9.

[9] Griffin J, Terry BE, Ray TL, et al. Comparison of end-tidal and transcutaneous measures of carbon dioxide during general anaesthesia in severely obese adults. Br J Anaesth 2003;91:498–501.

[10] Tobias JD. Noninvasive carbon dioxide monitoring during one-lung ventilation: end-tidal versus transcutaneous techniques. J Cardiothorac Vasc Anesth 2003;17:306–8.

[11] Ahrens T. Monitoring carbon dioxide in critical care: the newest vital sign? Crit Care Nurs Clin North Am 2004;16:445–51.

[12] Shoemaker W, Belzberg H, Wo C, et al. Multicenter study of noninvasive monitoring systems as alternative to invasive monitoring of acutely ill emergency patients. Chest 1998;114:1643–52.

[13] Linde Medical Sensors product information. Available at: http://www.linde-ms.ch. Accessed August 12, 2005.

[14] Masimo Corporation product information. Available at: http://www.masimo.com/products/tosca.htm. Accessed August 12, 2005.

[15] Sanders M, Kern NB, Constantino JP, et al. Accuracy of end-tidal and transcutaneous PCO$_2$ monitoring during sleep. Chest 1994;106:472–83.

[16] Clark JS, Voterri B, Ariagno RL, et al. Noninvasive assessment of blood gases. Am Rev Respir Dis 1992; 145:220–32.

[17] Capovilla J, VanCouwenberghe C, Miller W. Noninvasive blood gas monitoring. Crit Care Nurs Q 2000; 23:79–86.

ELSEVIER
SAUNDERS

Crit Care Nurs Clin N Am 18 (2006) 217–225

CRITICAL CARE
NURSING CLINICS
OF NORTH AMERICA

End-Tidal Carbon Dioxide Monitoring: A VITAL Sign Worth Watching

Karen Zwerneman, MSN, RN, CCRN

Neurology, Vasular, & Renal Services, Baylor University Medical Center, 3500 Gaston Avenue, Dallas, TX 75228, USA

What is capnography and why should this technology be monitored? Over the past 10 years, monitoring critical care patients with continuous pulse oximetry has become a practice standard for respiratory care; however, pulse oximetry is limited to providing information on oxygenation only; it tells nothing about the patient's ventilatory status [1]. Capnography, or the measurement of exhaled carbon dioxide (CO_2), provides feedback on alveolar ventilation. The CO_2 in exhaled gas is the product of three respiratory components: alveolar ventilation, transport, and pulmonary perfusion [2,3]. Capnography, in addition to pulse oximetry and other measures, provides the critical care clinician with complementary patient management information.

End-tidal CO_2 ($P_{ET}CO_2$) is the partial pressure of CO_2 present in the airway at the end of expiration. In intubated or spontaneously breathing patients, $P_{ET}CO_2$ can be continuously measured using several techniques: capnometry is the numeric (quantitative) measure of the CO_2 concentration in the airway throughout the ventilatory cycle; capnography is the numeric measure accompanied by the graphic display of the exhalation waveform over time (qualitative display); a capnogram is the waveform itself; and capnometers or capnographs are the machines used to measure levels of CO_2 in the airway [4,5].

Capnography is beneficial for monitoring ventilator status, warning of airway leaks and ventilatory circuit disconnections, estimating pulmonary dead space, and confirming proper endotracheal tube

(ETT) placement. Capnography also helps to diagnose certain medical conditions, make treatment decisions, assess hypoventilation during procedural sedation, evaluate the adequacy of chest compressions, and predict survival in cardiac arrest [5–7].

Why is the CO_2 level already available on measures of arterial blood gases (ABGs) not used to provide the same information? The CO_2 from ABGs provides only a numeric value. Would a clinician treat a heart rate alone without analyzing the corresponding EKG waveform? ABGs are a standard monitoring tool but are not continuous. Analysis of a capnogram over time provides information that a single CO_2 reading cannot. $P_{ET}CO_2$ values are affected by the matching of ventilation in the lungs with the perfusion of the pulmonary capillaries and are not strictly regulated by the patient's ventilatory status, as are arterial CO_2 (P_aCO_2) levels [2,5,8]. Using capnography as a supplementary tool provides an early warning sign in identifying trends in ventilation over time [8].

This article describes the uses of capnography in acute care settings, reviews the characteristics and treatment goals for normal and abnormal capnography waveforms, and illustrates how capnography can improve current practice.

Pathophysiology

CO_2 is produced as an end product of aerobic metabolism and oxygen use by the cells. During inspiration, air that contains minimal CO_2 is drawn into the alveoli and dilutes the CO_2 present in the functional residual capacities of the lung. At the same

E-mail address: karenz@baylorhealth.edu

time, as the CO_2 increases within the cells, CO_2 diffuses into the tissue capillaries and is carried by the blood to the lungs. Mixed venous blood returns to the pulmonary capillaries with high levels of CO_2, and then diffuses from the pulmonary capillaries into the alveoli for elimination. CO_2 moves in high concentrations from the blood down a concentration gradient to the alveoli, requiring no active metabolic work. At the end of expiration when fresh air is no longer diluting alveolar air, just before the next breath is taken in, alveolar and pulmonary capillary blood CO_2 gas tensions are at their highest levels. PETCO$_2$ is measured by way of capnography at this point [2,9,10].

PETCO$_2$ is the concentration of CO_2 in exhaled gas at the end of exhalation [3]. The three principal determinants of PETCO$_2$ are CO_2 production by the body, pulmonary dead space, and minute ventilation ($\dot{V}_E$). A normal PETCO$_2$ is 30 to 43 mm Hg at sea level [4]. A normal PaCO$_2$ obtained from an ABG sample is 34 to 45 mm Hg. This PaCO$_2$ to PETCO$_2$ difference (gradient) is due to alveolar dead space resulting from ventilation, perfusion, and gas exchange in the lungs [2]. Capnography reflects alveolar ventilation because the readings come from exhaled alveolar gas, which provides information on pulmonary perfusion [1].

Capnography is an important continuous and noninvasive monitoring tool but is not meant to replace ABG analysis. The patient monitored with capnography may require fewer ABG samples, but when questions arise regarding capnography results or the patient's pulmonary status, ABGs should be done to evaluate pH and other variables [1]. PaCO$_2$ levels can be predicted from capnography levels only if the dead space and pulmonary blood flow are normal. On initiation of capnography, one ABG sample should be analyzed to note the PaCO$_2$ – PETCO$_2$ difference [11]. When the PaCO$_2$ – PETCO$_2$ value is carefully established and tracked in selected patients, capnometry may be useful in adjusting ventilation and in reducing the need for ABG analyses [5].

CO_2 is transported in the body in three ways: approximately 65% as bicarbonate ions; approximately 25% bound to blood proteins, especially hemoglobin; and the remainder dissolved in plasma. The CO_2 dissolved in plasma is the CO_2 that is measured as the partial pressure of CO_2 in ABG analysis [5]. The CO_2 present at the end of exhalation is the CO_2 measured as PETCO$_2$ in capnography [3].

Increased PaCO$_2$ to PETCO$_2$ differences (increased PaCO$_2$ – PETCO$_2$ gradients) are thought to be largely caused by a reduced cardiac output or maldistribution of pulmonary blood flow. When the pulmonary system does not receive adequate alveolar perfusion, CO_2 does not return as readily to the lungs, causing increased alveolar dead space and larger differences between ventilation and perfusion [12]. This ventilation/perfusion mismatch may also be due to microemboli in the lung, which would cause ventilated but not perfused alveoli [13].

PETCO$_2$ is more affected by a ventilation/perfusion ($\dot{V}/\dot{Q}$) mismatch than PaCO$_2$ values because the PETCO$_2$ reflects alveolar gas composition. In situations such as shock, hypovolemia, significant pulmonary embolism, or cardiac arrest, PETCO$_2$ levels decrease when blood cannot bring as much CO_2 from the tissues to the alveoli. Hypoperfusion of the tissues results in decreased production of CO_2 at the cellular level, which causes decreased PETCO$_2$ levels during periods of systemic hypoperfusion [10]. In other instances, the application of positive end-expiratory pressure, age, smoking, general anesthesia, and major systemic disease cause decreased PETCO$_2$ levels [5]. PaCO$_2$ may or may not be reduced to the same degree. In the presence of a normal capnography waveform whereby the PaCO$_2$ – PETCO$_2$ gradient increases, typically there is a decrease in pulmonary perfusion [1]. In the presence of decreased pulmonary perfusion, PETCO$_2$ may not accurately reflect partial pressure of CO_2 levels [10].

Capnography can provide helpful information about systemic blood flow. In situations in which systemic blood flow is decreased, blood flow to the lungs is also decreased. This decrease in alveolar blood flow while alveolar ventilation is unchanged produces a widened PaCO$_2$ – PETCO$_2$ gradient [14,15].

Arterial carbon dioxide—end-tidal carbon dioxide gradient

In normal lungs, exhaled CO_2 levels closely approximate PaCO$_2$ levels [12]. "Carbon dioxide is first exhaled from the anatomic dead spaces, which have nearly infinite ventilation-perfusion ($\dot{V}/\dot{Q}$) ratios. Gas then comes from low-resistance lung areas with relatively high $\dot{V}/\dot{Q}$ ratios and low carbon dioxide levels. Finally, high-resistance lung units with lower $\dot{V}/\dot{Q}$ ratios and the highest carbon dioxide levels are emptied" [5]. At the end of expiration, the maximum partial pressure of CO_2 (PETCO$_2$) occurs, correlating with PaCO$_2$ levels in normal lungs. When lungs are normal, alveolar ventilation is matched by alveolar perfusion, a term referred to as the $\dot{V}/\dot{Q}$ ratio. In healthy patients, so long as ventilation matches perfusion, the difference between PaCO$_2$ and PETCO$_2$

(PaCO$_2$ – PETCO$_2$ gradient) generally varies from 2 to 5 mm Hg, with PaCO$_2$ exceeding PETCO$_2$. This value is determined by subtracting the PETCO$_2$ value from the PaCO$_2$ value [2,5,10,12]. If this is not the case with a patient's readings, then there may be a problem with $\dot{V}/\dot{Q}$ mismatching or shunting [8].

The PaCO$_2$ – PETCO$_2$ gradient reflects the amount of dead space ventilation. A low gradient, or a minimal difference between the two values, represents an optimal $\dot{V}/\dot{Q}$ relationship. The PaCO$_2$ – PETCO$_2$ gradient increases in patients who have lung disease probably because of changes in ventilation or perfusion. The gradient may increase with shallow or irregular breathing patterns [2]. It can alert the nurse to mechanical problems with the ventilator, such as a circuit leak or disconnection, ETT cuff leak, or ventilator malfunction. An increased gradient may also warn of a kinked or partially occluded ETT, airway obstruction, or bronchospasm [3]. Any condition that reduces pulmonary blood flow relative to ventilation causes this gradient to increase [11].

An initial assessment of the PaCO$_2$ – PETCO$_2$ gradient should be established by taking an ABG sample when capnography is initiated. This gradient should be documented and then used to manage the patient [3,8,14]. Ahrens and colleagues [11] suggested that $\dot{V}_E$ should also be monitored to determine dead space ventilation. $\dot{V}_E$ is the amount of air (measured in liters per minute) determined by the respiratory rate multiplied by the tidal volume. When the $\dot{V}_E$ is constant, one can expect dead space to remain relatively constant. When dead space changes, the patient's respiratory rate increases. When the $\dot{V}_E$ increases, one can expect PETCO$_2$ levels to decrease; if not, an increase in dead space may be occurring. With these types of changes in $\dot{V}_E$, an ABG is indicated to reassess the PaCO$_2$. It should be remembered that the greater the difference between the PaCO$_2$ and the PETCO$_2$ levels, the more severe the disruption between pulmonary ventilation and pulmonary perfusion.

Certain patient conditions decrease perfusion in relation to ventilation, causing an increase in physiologic dead space. Physiologic dead space includes lung areas not actively involved in gas exchange [5]. This type of $\dot{V}/\dot{Q}$ mismatch is commonly seen in pulmonary emboli, whereby blood flow is diverted from the area of obstruction to other pulmonary blood vessels. A pulmonary embolus diminishes pulmonary blood flow to the area involved but does not affect alveolar ventilation. Ventilation increases in other areas in an attempt to match the increased perfusion. One of the first signs of a pulmonary embolus, therefore, is an increase in $\dot{V}_E$, which is the product of respiratory rate multiplied by tidal volume, or the amount of air exhaled in 1 minute [11,14]. The PaCO$_2$ – PETCO$_2$ gradient increases as the dead space increases. This increased dead space—a result of reduced pulmonary blood flow—can be detected with capnography, and this information can be an early indicator before performing other diagnostic testing for pulmonary emboli [11,12].

Capnography use in critical care

PETCO$_2$ monitoring has many clinical applications in the critical care environment, including verifying and maintaining correct ETT placement, evaluating the effectiveness of cardiopulmonary resuscitation (CPR) compressions and identifying the return of spontaneous circulation, monitoring continuously during procedural sedation and anesthesia, assessing $\dot{V}/\dot{Q}$ status, evaluating ventilation status during weaning and following extubation, validating end expiration during hemodynamic waveform analysis, and verifying feeding tube placement.

Capnography is an effective way to confirm placement of ETTs. ETTs are lifesaving devices but their incorrect placement can be lethal. Because CO$_2$ is exhaled through the trachea and not the esophagus, capnography can detect esophageal intubation and measures can be taken to correct the placement. In patients who have a spontaneous pulse, ETT verification with PETCO$_2$ measures has been reported at 100%, whereas in cardiac arrest situations, it is less sensitive [5,14]. Current ACLS guidelines recommend the use of capnography, capnometry, or colorimetric detectors to confirm ETT placement during code situations [16].

Capnometry is also useful in ensuring ETT placement during patient transports [5]. The continuous numeric (quantitative) and waveform (qualitative) indicators from capnography translate to quick evidence of ETT dislodgment, displacement, or obstructions [3,4,11,12]. In the hospital setting, tubes can be moved or pulled when the patient is traveling to diagnostic imaging, when being moved from bed to procedural table, when the patient is turned, or when the patient becomes combative [4]. A sudden drop in the PETCO$_2$ level may result from extubation, airway secretions, or a mucus plug obstructing the airway, whereas a low PETCO$_2$ level may result form a cuff leak around the ETT [5,9]. In a recent sentinel event report on ventilator-associated deaths and injuries, the JCAHO reported that a high percentage of deaths or injuries were related to malfunction or misuse of the ventilator alarm, tubing disconnection, and disconnected tracheal tube or ETT [14]. Capnography use has proved to be an invaluable tool for the early identification of a dislodged tube.

During CPR, the measurement of $P_{ET}CO_2$ has been used to optimize chest compressions. A trend of decreasing $P_{ET}CO_2$ values helps detect rescuer fatigue and reveals when to change rescuers to optimize compressions [5,14,17].

The relationship between $P_{ET}CO_2$ and cardiac output is strong, even during CPR [5]. "During cardiac arrest, cardiac output falls resulting in a decrease in pulmonary blood flow. This decrease in blood flow causes the lung to inadequately eliminate CO_2 in expired gas leading to a rapid drop in the $P_{ET}CO_2$ level. Once normal cardiac output and pulmonary blood flow are restored, with either cardiopulmonary resuscitation or the return of normal cardiac function, the lung eliminates CO_2" [9]. This increase in $P_{ET}CO_2$ signals the return of spontaneous circulation and a successful resuscitation [3,11,12,17,18].

Monitoring $P_{ET}CO_2$ during procedural sedation or anesthesia gives the clinician a continuous assessment of ventilation during procedures. It provides breath-to-breath information on ventilation and respiratory effort and may alert the anesthesiologist or certified registered nurse anesthetist to early detection of respiratory depression before pulse oximetry changes [7,11].

The relationship between P_aCO_2 and $P_{ET}CO_2$ and the ratio between dead space and tidal volume is well established. Research on using this information to detect pulmonary embolism is promising but incomplete [5]. A decreased $P_{ET}CO_2$ along with an increased $P_aCO_2 - P_{ET}CO_2$ gradient may be an early indicator of pulmonary embolism, but at this point in the research, detected emboli have to be fairly large ($\geq 25\%$ vascular occlusion) and emphysema has to be absent. $P_{ET}CO_2$ may be used, however, to initiate other forms of assessments to diagnose pulmonary emboli [5,12,18].

In assessing $\dot{V}/\dot{Q}$ status, the $P_aCO_2 - P_{ET}CO_2$ gradient may be used to determine the optimum level of positive end-expiratory pressure. A low gradient reveals optimal $\dot{V}/\dot{Q}$ measures, and whichever level of positive end-expiratory pressure that produces the lowest gradient is the level to use to ensure adequate pulmonary blood flow for gas exchange. Overdistending the alveoli causes a redistribution of pulmonary blood flow and a widening of the $P_aCO_2 - P_{ET}CO_2$ gradient [2,9].

$P_{ET}CO_2$ monitoring is beneficial when assessing ventilatory status during weaning and following extubation. A change in CO_2 production or elimination, whether sudden or gradual, may occur during routine patient activities such as suctioning, reposi-

tioning, a change in ventilatory support, nutritional supplementation, CPR, or neuromuscular blockade [10]. In recovery room settings, $P_{ET}CO_2$ monitoring provides early detection for laryngeal edema/laryngeal spasm, partial or total airway obstruction, and ineffective airway clearance [3,12,19].

Hemodynamic waveforms are most reliable when read at the end of expiration, which is the point just before the next breath is taken, when alveolar and pulmonary capillary blood CO_2 gas tensions are at the highest level. With the use of $P_{ET}CO_2$, end expiration is easily identified. Many ICU nurses use the benefit of capnography to help them interpret hemodynamic information [11,12,14,20].

Whenever a tube is placed in the lungs, it is accompanied by vigorous coughing in the conscious patient; however, in the unconscious patient, the sedated patient, or the anesthetized patient, this coughing reflex may not be present. Placement of a feeding tube into the lungs may not be recognized until the radiologist reports improper placement. Although capnography has been useful in assuring that the ETT is not in the lungs, results have been limited in assuring correct placement of small bowel feeding tubes [14]. Specific placement of these tubes in the stomach, duodenum, or jejunum is unconfirmed [12,21].

Capnography use in other settings

Capnography is also a useful monitoring tool in settings other than critical care units. In prehospital use with emergency medical systems and transport, capnography has been used to verify and revalidate correct ETT placement in this highly mobile environment, evaluate CPR efforts for effectiveness, quickly recognize the return of a spontaneous pulse, and predict outcomes of survival or death in prehospital CPR [4,14,17,22]. In the emergency department, capnography has also been used to determine the ventilatory status of patients who have pre-existing respiratory diseases, to monitor during procedural sedation, to assess cardiopulmonary status of trauma patients, to assess the effectiveness of therapeutic interventions, and to alert clinicians to respiratory depression. In procedural areas like the cardiac catheterization laboratory, the gastrointestinal laboratory, or the pulmonary laboratory, capnography has been used to identify hypoventilation due to procedural sedation and pain medication administration [7].

In anesthesia and postanesthesia care, clinicians are using capnography to monitor for apnea and airway obstructions. Periods of apnea not detected for up to 20 seconds by anesthesia providers were quickly noted with capnography [6,14]. In intubated patients transported to and from the operating room and ICU, a variability for $PaCO_2$ was found after transport when $PETCO_2$ was not used for monitoring during hand ventilation. In patients requiring tight control of $PaCO_2$, such as patients who have increased intracranial pressures or pulmonary hypertension, this may be a significant clinical finding [23]. In patients undergoing emergency trauma surgery, the $PaCO_2$ – $PETCO_2$ gradient has been identified as a predictor of mortality and an indicator of physiologic stability [13].

Capnography equipment

There are three types of capnography equipment: mainstream, sidestream, and microstream. Mainstream capnography is used in intubated patients. A heated sensor is placed in the airway circuit between the ETT and the ventilator tubing. The exhaled gas flows directly over the sensor, providing an almost instantaneous measurement of $PETCO_2$. Disadvantages of microstream capnography are the weight of the sensor (increasing the risk of accidental extubation), the additional dead space within the tubing, and contamination of the sensor with sputum because it is positioned inline with the airway [1,5].

Sidestream capnography may be used in intubated or nonintubated patients. A small tube is placed between the airway and the ventilator tubing, and a pump continuously aspirates a sample from the exhaled breath. Sidestream technology is very lightweight but may be obstructed by moisture or sputum in the sample line. In addition, because the sample must travel, time delays may occur in analysis [1,12].

Microstream capnography, like sidestream technology, may be used in intubated and nonintubated patients. It is the newest technology in capnography monitoring and uses small sampling ports, low flow

rates, and low volumes. Microstream capnography has a decreased risk of sensor occlusion and may be used with nasal cannulalike devices [1,4,5].

The normal capnography waveform

The capnography waveform, or capnogram, provides information about the patient's ventilatory status beyond the CO_2 numeric display (Fig. 1). The waveform is read from left to right and represents the CO_2 concentration during the respiratory cycle, with each wave representing a single respiratory cycle. The waveform elevates on expiration, representing the increased CO_2 concentration in the exhaled gas. The capnogram consists of four phases: baseline, expiratory upstroke, expiratory or alveolar plateau, and inspiratory downstroke. The horizontal axis reflects time, and the vertical axis reflects the concentration of exhaled CO_2 [8,9,24].

Learning to analyze $PETCO_2$ waveforms is no more difficult than learning EKG interpretation or hemodynamic waveform analysis, and to the trained observer, $PETCO_2$ waveforms provide more information than the numeric display alone. Clinicians appreciate how much is gained when they can analyze patients' EKG waveforms, evaluate their hemodynamic waveforms, and not base treatment decisions solely on the numeric display; the same can be said of $PETCO_2$ monitoring. The shape of this waveform provides an abundance of information about a patient's ventilatory status, and changes in the capnogram can immediately alert the clinician to hypoventilation, apnea, or a wealth of other ventilatory issues.

The initial segment of the waveform is the baseline near the beginning of exhalation (A; see Fig. 1). This position represents inspiration of CO_2-free gases and includes the first stages of exhalation in which gases in anatomic dead spaces remain free of CO_2 (A–B; see Fig. 1). Because this air does not participate in gas exchange, the $PETCO_2$ level stays flat, and the value should be zero unless rebreathing of

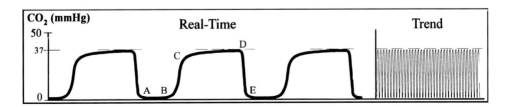

Fig. 1. Normal capnogram. A–B, baseline during inspiration; B–C, expiratory upstroke; C–D, expiratory or alveolar plateau; D, $PETCO_2$; D–E, inspiratory down-stroke. (Courtesy of Respironics Inc., Murryville, PA; with permission.)

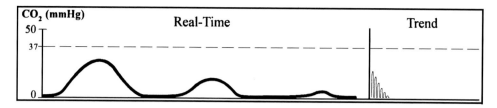

Fig. 2. ETT in the esophagus. (Courtesy of Respironics Inc., Murryville, PA; with permission.)

CO_2 is occurring because there is a malfunction in a ventilator circuit, the inspiratory flow is inadequate, or the expiratory time is insufficient [5,8–10].

The expiratory upstroke is the second phase of the waveform, representing a sudden increase from baseline as CO_2 is exhaled from the lungs (B–C; see Fig. 1). Gas from the intermediate airways begins to be exhaled from the lungs [10]. CO_2 concentration increases as CO_2 empties from rapidly exchanging alveolar spaces and mixes with dead space gas [8,9].

The third phase is the alveolar or expiratory plateau (C–D; see Fig. 1). It typically has a slight upward slope because of differences in alveolar emptying patterns. The plateau is determined by CO_2 concentrations in the exhaled gas, which are relatively constant because the gas is coming from lung units with similar $\dot{V}/\dot{Q}$ relationships [9]. The slight upward slope results because the sensor receives low levels of CO_2 gas from low-resistance areas of the lung with high $\dot{V}/\dot{Q}$ initially, and then receives gas from areas with progressively lower $\dot{V}/\dot{Q}$ and higher levels of CO_2 [5]. At the end of this plateau (D; see Fig. 1), the exhaled CO_2 concentration is highest, which is where $PETCO_2$ is measured. This position represents the exhalation from the most poorly ventilated alveolar units [8–10].

The fourth phase of the capnogram is the inspiratory downstroke (D–E; see Fig. 1). The rapidly descending limb represents inspiration and a return of CO_2 to a baseline of 0 mm Hg [9]. Inspiration rapidly

washes the expiratory gas away from the sensor, and the capnogram measures an inspired gas essentially devoid of CO_2 [8,10,14]. The cycle begins again with the next breath.

Why capnography is important: abnormal waveforms

When the ETT is correctly placed in the trachea, a normal capnogram can be seen; however, incorrect placement reveals a flat line and no waveform. A sudden loss of $PETCO_2$ to a waveform at baseline or near baseline indicates immediate danger because no respirations are detected (Fig. 2), which could be due to extubation, acute ventilator malfunction, tubing disconnection from the ventilator, a kinked or obstructed ETT, or cardiac arrest [5,9,10,12,24]. When no waveform is observed, one should immediately check the patient for airway obstruction or cardiac arrest, the ETT for disconnections, and the ventilator for malfunctions while hand ventilating the patient.

Sometimes the numeric $PETCO_2$ value changes but the waveform configuration remains constant. When this is the case, a change in ventilation, dead space, cardiac output, or metabolism has occurred [5]. When the value is rising, $PaCO_2$ may be rising with a reduction in alveolar ventilation. Gradual rising of the $PETCO_2$ value may be related to hyperthermia,

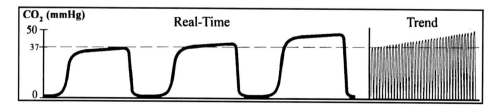

Fig. 3. Increasing $PETCO_2$ level. (Courtesy of Respironics Inc., Murryville, PA; with permission.)

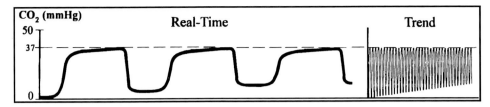

Fig. 4. Rising baseline. (Courtesy of Respironics Inc., Murryville, PA; with permission.)

hypoventilation, partial airway obstruction, CO_2 absorption from exogenous sources, sepsis, neuromuscular blockade, respiratory depressants, decreased alveolar ventilation, partial airway obstruction, or increases in CO_2 production from other sources (Fig. 3) [9,10,24].

A rising baseline reflects rebreathing of CO_2 (Fig. 4) [24], which may be due to ventilator causes such as inadequate inspiratory flow or insufficient expiratory time [5] or to exogenous sources such as sodium bicarbonate, body temperature, set respiratory rate, and set tidal volume [9]. A gradual rising of the baseline and $PETCO_2$ values (in combination) reflects rebreathing of exhaled gases due to additional dead space in the ventilator circuit or a defective exhalation valve [10].

Any condition that delays or restricts exhalation prolongs the upstroke (B–C; see Fig. 1) and may include a kinked ETT, a slow sidestream sampling rate, obstructive pulmonary disease, or bronchospasm [5].

A normal capnogram should have a plateau wave or a flattening of the waveform before the end of exhalation (C–D; see Fig. 1). When the slope continues to rise, there is inadequate alveolar ventilation, and bronchospasm, increased airway resistance, or increase in dead space is occurring [5,11]. In the asthmatic patient, these increases in airway resistance may be a way to track disease progression and tell whether bronchodilator therapy is working [5].

A small, poorly shaped expiratory waveform is observed when the patient's own respiratory muscles cannot support adequate ventilation during spontaneous breaths. During ventilator breaths, exhalation reveals an increase in $PETCO_2$, with a relatively normal waveform in a patient who does not have significant airway narrowing or copious secretions [1].

An abnormal biphasic capnogram has been noted in patients after single lung transplantation due to differing $\dot{V}/\dot{Q}$ ratios in each lung. The first peak represents expired CO_2 from the allograft lung, which has good $\dot{V}/\dot{Q}$ ratios, and the second peak, with a steeper plateau, represents the native lung that has mismatched $\dot{V}/\dot{Q}$ ratios [25].

A cleft in the alveolar or expiratory plateau ("curare" cleft) may be seen in patients who have an asynchronous spontaneous inspiration during mechanical ventilation (Fig. 5) [5,24]. This asynchronous spontaneous breath causes a dip in the expiratory plateau and may be associated with diaphragmatic contractions and inadequate inspiratory flow volumes. This dip may be seen in chemically paralyzed patients when they begin to regain muscle strength, indicating incomplete paralysis and the need for additional neuromuscular blockade [5,9,14].

A sudden decrease in $PETCO_2$ to a low but nonzero value occurs when full exhalation is not detected at the airway, which could be due to a partial disconnection in the tubing, a leak in the airway, partial obstruction due to secretions, or a fluid volume defi-

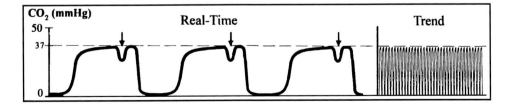

Fig. 5. Subsiding neuromuscular blockade or curare cleft. (Courtesy of Respironics Inc., Murryville, PA; with permission.)

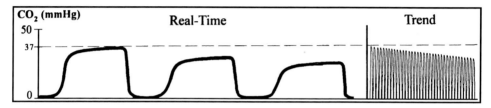

Fig. 6. Decreasing PETCO$_2$ level. (Courtesy of Respironics Inc., Murryville, PA; with permission.)

cit with sudden hypotension and massive blood loss. More gradual decreases in PETCO$_2$ may reflect decreased cardiac output, pulmonary embolism, decreasing body temperature, decreased contractility, or hypovolemia (Fig. 6) [9,10,14,24]. A sustained low PETCO$_2$ with a normal alveolar plateau configuration may represent chronic pulmonary diseases such as emphysema, bronchitis, asthma, and pneumonia. Actions should be aimed at increasing pulmonary perfusion, increasing fluid volume, increasing cardiac output and blood pressure, increasing body temperature, and assessing for pulmonary emboli [9]. A prolonged downstroke (D–E; see Fig. 1) is usually associated with a leak in the ventilator circuit or the ETT [5,14].

Summary

Not only should clinicians be aware of the benefits of capnography but they also should be using it in their practices. Learning to analyze a capnography waveform is as easy as monitoring an EKG waveform or a hemodynamic waveform, and the capnography waveform gives much more information than the numeric value alone.

The advantages of capnography in the critical care setting are immense. For patients who are intubated or nonintubated, the nurse can use the shape of the capnogram to determine airway obstructions and the need for suctioning (Fig. 7) [24]. With patients who

are asthmatic, the nurse can recognize airway narrowing and the efficacy of bronchodilator therapy and other interventions. When traveling to procedural areas, the nurse can confirm ETT placement for adequate ventilation during transport. During CPR, the code team can recognize when the clinician doing the chest compressions is tiring and then switch compressors and can quickly recognize the return of a spontaneous pulse. When weaning from mechanical ventilation, the nurse can tell whether the respiratory rate and tidal volume are sufficient by identifying trends with PETCO$_2$. During neuromuscular blockade, the nurse can identify when additional medications are needed by noting the shape of the waveform. During intubation, the nurse can tell immediately whether the ETT is correctly placed. During procedural sedation, the nurse can recognize apnea or hypoventilation more quickly and accurately than by respiratory rate or pulse oximetry alone. In the near future, the promising research aimed at predicting mortality in codes may also allow the nurse to stop futile resuscitations [26].

Without a clear understanding of the capnography waveform, however, this technology is just one more number to monitor and one more thing to document in the ever-technical critical care environment. To use capnography effectively, the critical care nurse must master normal and abnormal waveform patterns, use this knowledge to plan interventions with other critical care team members, and adjust these interventions based on the patient's response.

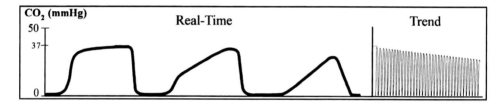

Fig. 7. Airway obstruction or obstruction in breathing circuit. (Courtesy of Respironics Inc., Murryville, PA; with permission.)

References

[1] Carroll P, Farquharson G. Using capnography effectively in critical care. AACN NTI News 2002;8:1–15.

[2] Kinney MR, Dunbar SB, Brooks-Brunn JA, et al. AACN clinical reference for critical care nursing. 4th edition. St. Louis (MO): Mosby; 1998.

[3] Sinclair S. Dispelling myths of capnography. Dimens Crit Care Nurs 1998;17(1):48–55.

[4] DeBoer S, Seaver M, Arndt K. Verification of endotracheal tube placement: a comparison of confirmation techniques and devices. J Emerg Nurs 2003;29(5):444–50.

[5] Frakes MA. Measuring end-tidal carbon dioxide: clinical applications and usefulness. Crit Care Nurse 2001;21(5):23–37.

[6] Soto RG, Fu ES, Vila HJ, et al. Capnography accurately detects apnea during monitored anesthesia care. Anesth Analg 2004;99(2):379–82.

[7] Oridion Medical. Oridion microstream capnography pocket guide. Danville (CA): Oridion Medical; 2000.

[8] Carroll P. Evolutions: capnography. RN 1999;62(5):69–71.

[9] LaValle TL, Perry AG. Capnography: assessing end-tidal CO_2 levels. Dimens Crit Care Nurs 1995;14(2):70–7.

[10] Good VS. Continuous end-tidal carbon dioxide monitoring. In: Lynn-McHale DJ, Carlson KK, editors. AACN procedural manual for critical care. 4th edition. Philadelphia: Saunders; 2001. p. 64–70.

[11] Ahrens T. Technology utilization in the cardiac surgical patient: SvO_2 and capnography monitoring. Crit Care Nurs Q 1998;21(1):24–40.

[12] Ahrens T, Wijeweera H, Ray S. Capnography: a key underutilized technology. Crit Care Nurs Clin North Am 1999;11(1):49–62.

[13] Tyburski JG, Collinge JD, Wilson RF, et al. End-tidal CO_2-derived values during emergency trauma surgery correlated with outcome: a prospective study. J Trauma 2002;53(4):738–43.

[14] Ahrens T, Sona C. Capnography application in acute and critical care. AACN Clin Issues 2003;14(2):123–32.

[15] Jin X, Weil MH, Tang W, et al. End-tidal carbon dioxide as a noninvasive indicator of cardiac index during circulatory shock. Crit Care Med 2000;28(7):2415–9.

[16] Cummins RO, editor. ACLS: principles and practice. Dallas (TX): American Heart Association; 2004.

[17] Cantineau JP, Lambert Y, Merckx P, et al. End-tidal carbon dioxide during cardiopulmonary resuscitation in humans presenting mostly with asystole: a predictor of outcome. Crit Care Med 1996;24(5):791–6.

[18] Weg SD, Surgenor JG. A new niche for end-tidal CO_2 in pulmonary embolism. Crit Care Med 2000;28(11):3752–4.

[19] Cook D, Meade M, Guyatt G, et al. Trials of miscellaneous interventions to wean from mechanical ventilation. Chest 2001;120(6):438S–44S.

[20] Bhavani-Shankar K, Philip JH. Defining segments and phases of time capnogram. Anesth Analg 2000;91(4):973–7.

[21] Burns SM, Carpenter R, Truwitt JD. Report on the development of a procedure to prevent placement of feeding tubes into the lungs using end-tidal CO_2 measurements. Crit Care Med 2001;29(5):936–9.

[22] Levine RL, Wayne MA, Miller CC. End-tidal carbon dioxide and outcome of out-of-hospital cardiac arrest. N Engl J Med 1997;337(5):301–6.

[23] Palmon SC, Liu M, Moore LE, et al. Capnography facilitates tight control of ventilation during transport. Crit Care Med 1996;24(4):608–11.

[24] Capnography: a reference handbook. Solar 8000M patient monitor operator's manual. Milwaukee (WI): GE Medical Systems Information Technologies; 2001. p. 23–32.

[25] Srinivasa V, Kodali BS, Hartigan PM. Evolving capnograms after single lung transplant. Anesth Analg 2004;98(5):1504.

[26] Tyburski JG, Carlin AM, Harvey EHS, et al. End-tidal CO_2-arterial CO_2 differences: a useful intraoperative mortality marker in trauma surgery. J Trauma 2003;55(5):892–7.

ELSEVIER
SAUNDERS

CRITICAL CARE
NURSING CLINICS
OF NORTH AMERICA

Crit Care Nurs Clin N Am 18 (2006) 227 – 241

Impact of Bispectral Index Monitoring on Sedation and Outcomes in Critically Ill Adults: a Case Series

Richard Arbour, RN, MSN, CCRN, CNRN

Albert Einstein Healthcare Network, 5501 Old York Road, Philadelphia, PA 19141-3211, USA

The "gold standard" for assessing stability of neurologic function remains the clinical neurologic evaluation; however, there are clinical situations in which the ability to perform an adequate neurologic examination is limited. One situation is neuromuscular blockade (NMB). In this instance, the critically ill patient may be awake and in pain but appear to be calm and anxiety- and pain-free. A second situation is deep sedation to facilitate controlled ventilation. In this instance, the critically ill patient may potentially experience hemodynamic and neuroendocrine consequences of acute severe pain and appear deeply sedated. A third situation is following loss of consciousness subsequent to structural or metabolic brain injury. In these and similar situations, electrophysiologic monitoring of the brain such as with the cortical electroencephalogram (EEG) is an effective means to directly assess stability of the central nervous system.

Physiologic basis for the electroencephalogram

Approximately 50% of metabolic activity of the brain is directed toward generating and conducting neuronal electrical activity, with the balance maintaining structural integrity of the cells. As such, alterations in metabolic stability or metabolic activity of the brain are reflected in the cortical EEG. At the most basic level, the cortical EEG reflects electrical activity in the cerebral cortex. Electrical activity measured and recorded at the cerebral cortex is modulated by multiple factors. First, electrical discharges from the thalamus are regulated by relative proportions of excitatory and inhibitory neuronal connections. Second, presynaptic neurotransmitter release facilitates nerve impulse generation and conduction. As defined, multiple energy-consuming steps must occur to maintain stable brain metabolism and stability of brain metabolism as reflected in the cortical EEG [1–5].

Brain injury, whether metabolic or structural, and variables including multiple drug therapies may affect cerebral metabolism and EEG activity. Pharmacologic agents affecting brain metabolism and the EEG include benzodiazepines, propofol, and barbiturate therapy. Opioids may affect EEG activity at higher doses when sedation occurs as a side effect of therapy [6,7]. In a dose-related manner and pursuant to appropriate therapeutic goals, changes in EEG frequency, EEG amplitude, and EEG suppression may be produced [1,2,6]. With regard to monitoring drug therapy and clinical end points, EEG has long been used in monitoring clinical situations including drug-induced coma and effectiveness of anticonvulsant therapy [1,2].

Other potential clinical applications for EEG-based monitoring include use in monitoring sedation in critically ill adults in selected cases. Large-scale use of diagnostic EEG technology to monitor sedation in intensive care units is impractical. Limitations include size of monitoring technology, electrode application and maintenance, and difficulty interpreting the volume of information obtained [2,8,9]. One

E-mail address: richnrs@aol.com

area in which EEG-based technology is under study is in monitoring the level of sedation in critically ill patients. After administration of sedative and opioid analgesic agents in a dose-related manner, characteristic changes occur; specifically, a dose-dependent decrease in the level of consciousness, which in turn correlates with characteristic changes in EEG activity. Dose-dependent changes in EEG activity that occur with administration of sedative-hypnotic, opioid, or anesthetic agents include augmentation of beta (high-frequency) activity, which correlates with initial stages of sedation such as amnesia or anxiolysis. Further dose increases produce additional decreases in the level of consciousness and in EEG changes including increased proportion of slow-wave (delta and theta) activity. High-dose therapy with agents such as barbiturates or propofol can produce varying degrees of EEG suppression that correlate with a state of deep unconsciousness [1,2,6].

Relationship between the bispectral index and the electroencephalogram

In terms of monitoring drug therapy and therapeutic end points, EEG has long been used to study drug effects on the brain and to monitor clinical states such as barbiturate coma. A possible emerging technology to monitor level of sedation in critically ill patients is a derived EEG parameter, the bispectral index (BIS). The BIS was initially studied and used in the operating room setting. This parameter was designed to assess responses to sedation and anesthesia but is being used in some settings for monitoring sedation in critically ill adults. BIS determination begins with acquisition of EEG data that is passed through multiple processing steps, producing the specific BIS value. The BIS value is displayed on a linear (0–100) scale and shows varying correlation with clinical assessment of sedation. A BIS value approaching 100 typically corresponds with an awake state. A BIS value at or near 0 indicates minimal or no brain activity. Additional clinical end points and corresponding BIS values are found on a continuum between these extremes and are well described in the professional literature [1,2,7,9]. The BIS is a derived EEG parameter, and under normal conditions, EEG activity can change in response to stimulation and altered metabolic states such as cerebral ischemia, neurologic injury, and hypothermia. These alterations in cerebral physiology may also be reflected in the BIS value [1–3,10]. Secondary parameters available during BIS monitoring include electromyographic (EMG) activity. EMG activity is typically

high frequency in nature and may produce an elevation of the BIS value independent of hypnotic state [1,2,7,9]. The suppression ratio represents the percentage of suppressed EEG activity within the previous 63 seconds of EEG data. For example, if 25% of the EEG activity within the previous 63-second data sample is suppressed, then the suppression ratio is 25. If there is total EEG suppression consequent to catastrophic brain injury or significant overdosing of barbiturate therapy, then the suppression ratio may approach 100 [1,2,7,11]. A complete discussion of BIS derivation from the EEG is beyond the scope of this article. For a comprehensive discussion of BIS derivation, the reader is referred to any of the excellent references on this topic [1,2,7,9,11].

Sedation issues in adult critical care

Multiple sedation issues are encountered in critically ill adults. One issue is risk of undersedation, with attendant mobilization of physiologic stress, unrelieved agitation, and potential for awareness during NMB [7,8]. A second risk is oversedation, with attendant risks including interference with an adequate neurologic examination and hemodynamic compromise. Risks of oversedation also include prolonged recovery of consciousness and increased ventilator days with extended ICU length of stay [7,8]. For these reasons, sedation of critically ill adults is optimally managed with close monitoring and titration of therapy using a protocol-driven approach to care. Protocol-directed sedation practice has been shown to decrease ICU length of stay and improve outcomes in critically ill patients [12–14].

In clinical practice, optimal monitoring to navigate between the extremes of over- and undersedation is paramount and integral to a research-based and protocol-driven approach to sedation/analgesia management. Sedation assessment is generally done by means of clinical assessment tools. In practice, these assessment tools typically assign a numeric value on a linear scale to a specific set of physical/behavioral symptoms. Clinical assessment tools such as the Sedation-Agitation Scale (SAS),the Motor Activity Assessment Scale, and the Ramsay Sedation Scale have been studied and used in practice [15]. Clinical assessment of level of sedation and analgesia is optimal. There are limited circumstances in which clinical assessment may be inadequate to gauge level of sedation and analgesia. These circumstances include deep sedation/analgesia, drug-induced coma, and NMB. In these circumstances, clinical evaluation of cerebral function is significantly compromised and the use of EEG-based monitoring may potentially have a role in sedation practice.

Literature review

EEG-based monitoring with the BIS has been studied to evaluate its effectiveness in assessing sedation in critically ill patients. Multiple reports and studies have been published that illustrate its potential and some of its limits in terms of providing feedback on stability of brain function related to therapeutic decisions or clinical changes. A recent study by Riker and colleagues [16] compared the BIS and its corresponding suppression ratio with level of burst suppression on the diagnostic EEG. From 12 patients, 62 patient-days of data were obtained. Within the study sample, the investigators found strong correlation between BIS value, suppression ratio, and number of bursts per minute as monitored by diagnostic EEG during drug-induced coma using barbiturate therapy.

Fabregas and colleagues [17] studied whether BIS monitoring could yield additional information regarding the probability of recovery of consciousness in brain-injured patients. The investigators found statistically significant differences between groups of patients who did and did not recover consciousness with respect to BIS values and their corresponding secondary parameters and Glasgow Coma Scale scores. The investigators concluded that the BIS might potentially add to the body of clinical data and help predict probability of recovery of consciousness after withdrawal from sedation following brain injury.

A study by Vivien and colleagues [18] evaluated the impact of EMG activity on BIS values in a series of patients who received sedation/analgesia sufficient to achieve an SAS score of 1 (unarousable). The investigators found that administration of NMB resulted in a significant decline in BIS values, suggesting that even in deeply sedated patients, high EMG activity remains a significant potential limitation when using BIS monitoring for critically ill patients.

Gill and colleagues [19] studied the effectiveness of BIS technology in monitoring sedation in an emergency department (ED) setting. The investigators hypothesized that BIS values would correlate with clinical assessment of sedation in this patient population. The visual analog scale was used by data collection personnel who were blinded to BIS values. BIS values were later paired with corresponding visual analog scale scores. The investigators found only fair correlation between the BIS and clinical assessment of sedation. Based on the results from this study sample, the BIS was not shown to be effective in monitoring sedation adequacy in intubated ED patients.

A recent study by Deogaonkar and coworkers [20] evaluated correlation between BIS values and clinical assessment of sedation in brain-injured patients. The investigators found a statistically significant correlation between BIS values and clinical assessment of sedation and level of consciousness. Within the study sample, the investigators found stronger correlation between the BIS and clinical assessment using the newer version of BIS technology (BIS A-2000XP) and concluded that the BIS has potential as an adjunctive monitoring tool in patients following brain injury.

Kim and colleagues [21] investigated the effects of environmental noise on the BIS during sedation with propofol. The effects of ambient noise levels on cerebral arousal are significant when one considers the generally high decibel levels encountered in critical care units. The cerebral arousal resulting from environmental noise may possibly increase sedative requirements. The investigators found a temporal relationship between elevations in BIS values and controlled applications of noise from an external source. This effect was more pronounced at lighter levels of sedation (BIS value of 80), with propofol being the agent used.

Additional study of correlation between the BIS and clinical assessment of sedation was undertaken by Mondello and coworkers [22]. The investigators obtained 980 paired observations and found statistically significant correlations between the BIS and the Ramsay Sedation Scale.

Correlation between the BIS and the Comfort score was investigated by Courtman and colleagues [23]. The researchers found moderate correlation between BIS values and Comfort scores in critically ill children. This result is generally consistent with available literature that illustrates varying degrees of correlation between BIS values and clinical assessment of sedation.

Three case reports illustrate the potential sensitivity of the BIS to the instability of cerebral physiology. In the first case, the BIS was used for anesthesia management during cardiac anesthesia. During the coronary bypass graft procedure, profound hypotension occurred, with concurrent dramatic decline in BIS value. BIS values returned to baseline on restoration of cerebral perfusion. Limitations of the BIS for assessing periods of cerebral ischemia include the fact that BIS monitoring reflects EEG activity in the left or the right frontal-temporal montage. As such, it is nonspecific to location of cerebral instability and reflects global changes in cerebral physiology. The BIS demonstrated sensitivity to compromised cerebral perfusion in this setting [24]. In the second case, BIS monitoring was used following off-pump coronary bypass surgery. In the immediate postoperative period, the patient experienced significant hemorrhage followed by cardiac arrest. Progressive hypotension and pulseless electrical activity was accompanied by concurrent decline in BIS values. BIS values increased with effective cardiac compressions and successful resuscitation [25]. In the third case, BIS monitoring was used to monitor sedation in an elderly patient receiving sufantanil and midazolam. During one period, BIS values ranged from 40 to 52. Serum glucose was measured, and the patient was found to be profoundly hypoglycemic. Dextrose 30% was administered by infusion, and within minutes, rapid elevation of BIS values occurred, ranging from 59 to 82. Occurrence of EEG changes consequent to severe hypoglycemia, including slow-wave activity and varying degrees of EEG suppression, is well documented. Because BIS values are sensitive to changes in cerebral physiology, the BIS has potential in some patients to provide an early indication of brain instability, facilitating earlier intervention [26].

Simmonds and colleagues [27] researched sedation assessment using the SAS and the BIS. In this study, the researchers found positive correlation between the BIS as an EEG-based monitoring tool and clinical assessment of sedation. Positive correlation between the BIS and clinical assessment of sedation also matches the author's clinical experience in sedation monitoring using the BIS and clinical assessment tools.

In summary, review of the literature reveals several things. First, evidence of varying degrees of correlation between the BIS and clinical assessment of sedation is documented. Clinical assessment is and should remain the gold standard for assessing the level of sedation and brain function; however, there are circumstances in which the ability to perform optimal clinical assessment of sedation may be compromised. In clinical situations such as NMB and deep sedation/analgesia, EEG-based monitoring may have a role in monitoring and management of drug therapy. Second, as an EEG-based parameter, the BIS is sensitive to instability or compromise of cerebral physiology relative to electrode location. It is well documented that EEG changes including varying levels of EEG suppression and changes in EEG frequencies occur in response to metabolic or structural brain injury [2]. The BIS, however is not specific to location or type of brain injury. As such, its utility may be limited to providing an early warning of occurrence or progression in metabolic or structural brain injury relative to electrode location. A number of studies exist that demonstrate varying degrees of correlation between the BIS and clinical assessment of sedation. In addition, many case reports have been published that illustrate BIS sensitivity to metabolic or structural brain injury. EMG activity remains a significant potential confounding factor when interpreting BIS values. As such, BIS values should be interpreted within the context of clinical goals of therapy and with monitoring EMG as a secondary parameter. Clinical experience and published work using BIS technology clearly support further study. Studies that have evaluated outcomes between groups of patients (one group monitored with the BIS plus clinical assessment and a second group monitored with clinical assessment alone) to determine level of sedation and guide therapy are not extensive. Outcomes related to sedation include number of ventilator days, ICU length of stay, and additional costs. Additional ventilator and ICU days add significantly to financial costs of health care in acute care settings [28].

Sedation practices have been identified as significantly impacting such outcomes as ventilator days and ICU length of stay [7,12–15]. The potential impact of BIS monitoring on sedation outcomes was investigated by the author. Additional length of ICU stay and increased number of ventilator days are associated with increased morbidity including ventilator-associated pneumonia, airway injury, and potential risk of neurologic and neuropsychiatric complications in the critically ill patient. Of the multiple factors impacting length of ICU stay and number of ventilator days, optimal sedation management has significant potential to positively affect outcomes. Specific patient outcomes that may be improved by optimal sedation practices include times to extubation, decreased use of NMB, and ICU length of stay.

Patients, methods, and results

Patients

This case series evaluated 15 patients who required controlled-ventilation sedation/analgesia with and without NMB therapy. All patients met inclusion criteria, including absence of structural or metabolic brain injury such as severe renal/hepatic encephalopathic states, hypoxic/ischemic brain injury, or severe hypoxemia/hypercapnia causing compromised level of consciousness. Additional inclusion criteria included negative history of brain trauma and ischemic or hemorrhagic stroke. Because the BIS was developed based, in part, on an extensive database of normal EEG tracings, optimal evaluation of BIS monitoring in this case series was considered most appropriate to include patients who had intact neurologic function. As such, EEG-based monitoring using the BIS would be a more accurate reflection of the effects of sedative and analgesic agents on the uninjured brain. Determining degree of correlation between the BIS and clinical assessment of sedation was also facilitated by including patients who had intact neurologic function. As part of standard pharmacologic therapy for sedation/analgesic and NMB management, patients were prescribed (as indicated) opioid analgesics and sedative hypnotics, with and without NMB agents to attain appropriate end points as determined by clinical goals.

Methods

Patients meeting inclusion criteria received drug therapy using opioid and sedative/hypnotic, with and without NMB agents as indicated for specific clinical goals. These goals included synchrony with controlled ventilation, control of agitation, and appropriate sedation and analgesia during NMB and sedation/anxiolysis. BIS electrodes were placed using the right or the left frontal-temporal montage for EEG signal acquisition. Patients receiving therapy with sedative/hypnotic or opioid agents (without NMB) were monitored using BIS and clinical assessment of sedation level. In this subset of patients, therapeutic decisions were made primarily based on clinical assessment findings. The degree of correlation between the BIS value and clinical assessment of sedation was determined using the SAS.

Patients receiving NMB therapy concurrent with sedation/analgesia to facilitate ventilator management or to control life-threatening agitation were monitored using the BIS. In this subset of patients, the BIS was used as an adjunct to clinical assessment. By providing information unavailable by clinical examination, the BIS assisted in titration of drug therapy. To provide a basis for comparison, data were collected as part of quality assurance initiatives to establish baselines for clinical outcomes. Data included length of intubation/ventilation following withdrawal of sedation, duration of NMB, and incidence of awareness while receiving NMB. Throughout the evaluation of this case series, the question "Was BIS monitoring decisive in managing drug therapy?" was asked. Over the course of this case series, the team had the opportunity to use two versions of the BIS: BIS A-2000 and BIS A-2000XP.

Results

BIS monitoring was decisive in therapeutic decisions regarding sedation/analgesia and NMB in 9 of 15 patients in this series. In the remaining 6 patients, the BIS values that were obtained showed varying degrees of positive correlation with clinical assessment of sedation. The most significant potential benefit associated with BIS monitoring in this series was noted with BIS use in patients receiving NMB. In this subset of patients, BIS provided information unavailable by clinical assessment tools for level of sedation/cerebral arousal. Clinical results with basic descriptions of diagnosis, outcomes, and drug therapy are found in Table 1.

Case reports: bispectral index monitoring with neuromuscular blockade

Case 1

A 59-year-old patient who had a history of severe chronic obstructive pulmonary disease experienced progressive shortness of breath at home and was brought to the ED by emergency medical services. ED evaluation showed severe respiratory distress and hypercapnic respiratory failure. Endotracheal intubation was performed to facilitate ventilation and oxygenation. Despite aggressive sedation, the patient remained out of phase with controlled ventilation and received NMB. Following ICU admission and stabilization, NMB was weaned off for neurologic evaluation. The patient became progressively agitated and dys-synchronous with controlled ventilation. BIS monitoring was initiated and correlated with clinical assessment of arousal state. Aggressive sedation/analgesia was administered using lorazepam and fentanyl, which was effective only in the short-term as evidenced by periods of breakthrough agitation. Propofol was administered as a low-dose infusion, with dramatic decline in level of consciousness and BIS value. Clinical assessment was similar at BIS values of 10 and 45. Propofol and lorazepam were titrated back, allowing elevation in BIS value to between 40 and 50. This BIS value correlated with good patient–ventilator interface. In this patient, BIS monitoring allowed titration in real-time of sedative/hypnotic agents as an adjunct to clinical assessment and helped avoid NMB use.

Table 1

Case series illustrating potential benefit of bispectral index monitoring and correlation with clinical assessment of sedation when incorporated into practice in patients in whom clinical assessment is equivocal or compromised, such as during deep sedation/analgesia and neuromuscular blockade

Patient	Age (y)	Diagnosis	Sedative agent	Analgesic agent	NMB agent	NMB duration	BIS A-2000 versus BIS A-2000XP	BIS monitoring decisive in management?	Duration of NMB following start of BIS monitoring	Number of observations (BIS/SAS)[a]
1	59	COPD exacerbation	Lorazepam and propofol	Fentanyl	Cisatracurium/ vecuronium	7 h	A-2000	Yes, facilitated earlier withdrawal of NMB, tracked periods of oversedation following initiation of propofol, and showed correlation with clinical assessment of sedation	N/A, facilitated titration of sedation/analgesia and avoidance of NMB	13
2	58	Respiratory failure, severe PCP pneumonia, end-stage HIV infection	Lorazepam	Fentanyl	Cisatracurium	67.5 h	A-2000	Yes, facilitated earlier withdrawal of NMB and showed correlation with clinical assessment	2.5 h	10
3	58	Epiglottitis	Lorazepam	Morphine	Cisatracurium	12 h	A-2000	Yes, facilitated earlier withdrawal of NMB, avoided over/under sedation, and identified patient as at risk for awareness and pain while paralyzed	2 h	14
4	86	Pneumonia, respiratory failure	Lorazepam	N/A	N/A	N/A	A-2000	No, showed correlation with clinical assessment, adjunct to clinical assessment	N/A	7
5	45	Exacerbation of COPD, progressive respiratory failure	Lorazepam, midazolam	Ketorolac	N/A	N/A	A-2000	No, assessed correlation with clinical examination	N/A	26
6	33	Severe ETOH withdrawal, seizures	Lorazepam	Fentanyl	N/A	N/A	A-2000	No, assessed correlation with clinical examination	N/A	14

7	60	Respiratory failure secondary to severe COPD	Lorazepam	Morphine	N/A	N/A	A-2000	No, tracked recovery from long-term sedation, assessed correlation	N/A	9
8	39	End-stage liver disease, bleeding esophageal varices	Midazolam	N/A	Cisatracurium	15 h	A-2000	No, tracked recovery, assessed correlation with clinical assessment	N/A	41
9	26	PCP pneumonia, respiratory failure	Lorazepam, midazolam	Fentanyl	Cisatracurium	141 h	A-2000	Yes, guided sedation and analgesia therapy during NMB; enabled lower vasopressor dosing related to reduced sedation/analgesia dosing	N/A, guided therapy during NMB	N/A
10	69	Interstitial pneumonia, ARDS	Midazolam	Fentanyl	Cisatracurium	69 h	A-2000	Yes, identified significant EEG suppression (initial indication of severe neurologic injury), confirmed by diagnostic EEG; altered direction of care	1 h	N/A, patient had severe brain injury
11	35	Pneumonia, shock	Lorazepam, midazolam	Fentanyl.	Cisatracurium	N/A, patient died in ICU	A-2000XP	Yes, facilitated drug titration, changes in drug therapy during NMB	57 h until patient expired; used to titrate/change therapy while patient received NMB	N/A
12	54	ETOH withdrawal, seizures, severe agitation	Midazolam	Fentanyl	Cisatracurium	13 h	A-2000XP	Yes, facilitated earlier withdrawal of NMB and showed correlation between BIS and clinical assessment	2 h	7
13	33	Status asthmaticus, respiratory failure	Lorazepam, midazolam	Fentanyl	Cisatracurium, vecuronium	3 h	A-2000XP	During NMB only, titration of therapy, helped to avoid extremes of over/under sedation	3 h	15

(continued on next page)

234   ARBOUR

Table 1 (*continued*)

Patient	Age (y)	Diagnosis	Sedative agent	Analgesic agent	NMB agent	NMB duration	BIS A-2000 versus BIS A-2000XP	BIS monitoring decisive in management?	Duration of NMB following start of BIS monitoring	Number of observations (BIS/SAS)[a]
14	57	HIV infection, severe respiratory failure	Lorazepam	Fentanyl	Cisatracurium	120 h	A-2000XP	Yes, facilitated earlier withdrawal of NMB therapy, identified potential awareness and pain during NMB; with removal of NMB, evolving intra-abdominal process was identified and treated	2 h	12
15	66	Bronchogenic lung cancer, respiratory distress	Lorazepam	Morphine	Cisatracurium	6.5 h	A-2000XP	Yes, facilitated earlier withdrawal of NMB, identified cerebral arousal associated with painful procedure during NMB	4.5 h	18

Abbreviations: ARDS, acute respiratory distress syndrome; COPD, chronic obstructive pulmonary disease; ETOH, alcohol; N/A not applicable; PCP, *Pneumocystis carinii* pneumonia.

[a] Number of paired observations (BIS/SAS) obtained using BIS A-2000 in this series totaled 134. Number of paired observations (BIS/SAS) obtained using BIS A-2000XP in this series totaled 52.

Case 2

A 58-year-old patient who had a history of HIV infection and *Pneumocystis carinii* pneumonia (PCP) was admitted to the ICU and intubated for management of respiratory failure. Sedation/analgesia was managed using lorazepam and fentanyl. Ventilator dys-synchrony persisted despite aggressive sedative/opioid dosing. NMB was initiated using cisatracurium. Following initiation of BIS monitoring, the patient was noted to have a potential cerebral arousal state related to noxious stimulation. Supplemental dosing with fentanyl caused a decrease in the BIS value and blunted response to painful stimulation. NMB was weaned off 2.5 hours following initiation of BIS monitoring. In this patient, BIS-guided sedation and analgesia facilitated withdrawal of NMB and consequent recovery of ability to perform an adequate clinical evaluation of sedation end points and neurologic status.

Case 3

A 58-year-old patient who had a history of hypertension (controlled with β-blocker and calcium channel blocker therapy) and diabetes mellitus (controlled with oral hypoglycemic agents) presented to the ED with excessive salivation and speech described as a "whisper." Direct laryngoscopic examination revealed severe soft tissue swelling and critical airway narrowing. Elective endotracheal intubation was performed for airway protection. Following intubation, the patient was dys-synchronous with ventilation, agitated and combative, and refractory to sedation/analgesic administration as titrated to that point in time. NMB was initiated for control of agitation and combativeness and to maintain the airway. Following ICU admission, BIS monitoring was initiated and revealed potential awareness during NMB. Aggressive weight-based dosing of lorazepam and morphine was begun, which resulted in a decline in BIS value to between 50 and 60. After stabilization, NMB was weaned off permanently, which preserved ability to assess level of sedation and neurologic status by clinical assessment. Clinical assessment of sedation correlated with BIS value. The patient was weaned and extubated and transferred out of the ICU the following day, with discharge to home the next day. In this case, the BIS facilitated withdrawal of NMB, earlier extubation, and ICU discharge. Without EEG-based monitoring during NMB, the patient was at risk for over- or undersedation.

Case 9

Progressive respiratory failure in a 26-year-old patient who had a history of advanced HIV infection and PCP pneumonia necessitated endotracheal intubation and controlled ventilation. The patient received sedation/analgesia and subsequently NMB for ventilator management. Hemodynamic instability consequent to sepsis required norepinephrine for vasopressor support. In this patient, clinical assessment of sedation was not possible due to NMB use. BIS monitoring was initiated and initially revealed low BIS values (30–50). As such, sedation/analgesia was titrated back as indicated to maintain BIS values between 50 and 55 during NMB. Lower dosing of sedation/analgesia facilitated decreased norepinephrine dosing requirements. In this patient, BIS monitoring identified oversedation during NMB and enabled appropriate downward titration of sedative/analgesic agents followed by decreased vasopressor requirements.

Case 10

A 69-year-old patient was admitted to the ICU with community-acquired pneumonia. Progressive increases in oxygen requirements and respiratory failure were treated with oxygen by face mask, non-invasive positive-pressure ventilation, and ultimately endotracheal intubation/controlled ventilation. Midazolam and fentanyl were used for sedation and analgesia needs. The patient progressed to acute respiratory distress syndrome (ARDS) and required nonphysiologic ventilation modes including pressure control inverse ratio ventilation to maintain oxygenation. To facilitate controlled ventilation, NMB was used. The patient had unstable cardiopulmonary function such that withdrawal of NMB for clinical neurologic evaluation was not tolerated. While receiving NMB, BIS monitoring was initiated. The dramatically low BIS value (15–20) and a high suppression ratio were surprising findings. NMB was weaned off to facilitate neurologic assessment. The patient was minimally responsive; sedative/analgesic agents were also weaned off, with no subsequent change in the clinical assessment. Bedside neurologic evaluation including diagnostic EEG was done, which revealed irreversible and severe anoxic/ischemic brain injury. The family was notified and returned to the hospital for a family conference. When presented with this new information, the family made a decision for a "do not resuscitate" status, and the patient died peacefully within 36 hours. In this patient, EEG-based monitoring with the BIS provided an initial indication of potentially severe brain injury. This indication, which was not available by clinical assessment, ultimately led to a significant and appropriate change in direction of care.

Case 11

A 35-year-old patient was admitted to the ICU with pneumonia and developed septic shock during his ICU course. Severe respiratory failure required intubation and controlled ventilation. Lorazepam, midazolam, and fentanyl were used for initial management of anxiety and pain and to facilitate controlled ventilation. Respiratory failure progressed to acute respiratory distress syndrome, requiring nonphysiologic ventilation modes and subsequently NMB to facilitate ventilation. BIS monitoring was initiated during NMB and facilitated titration and change of sedative/analgesic agents in real-time when clinical assessment of sedation was not possible.

Case 12

A 54-year-old patient was admitted to the ICU following endotracheal intubation to manage alcohol withdrawal, severe agitation, and seizure activity. Severe agitation persisted despite escalating doses of sedative and analgesic agents. NMB was initiated to maintain synchrony with ventilation and to control breakthrough agitation/combativeness during sedative/opioid titration. BIS monitoring was initiated while in the ICU and revealed BIS values above 65, which increased further following endotracheal suctioning. Additional bolus doses of fentanyl and midazolam were administered, decreasing the BIS value to between 55 and 60. NMB was weaned off at this point, and the patient was responsive to noxious stimulation but no longer agitated. Sedative/analgesic agents were weaned down based on clinical assessment findings. The patient was extubated by early afternoon and transferred out of the ICU the following day. The BIS provided decisive information in this case by revealing potential awareness and pain while paralyzed, a potential cause of the patient's agitation before NMB was initiated. Without EEG-based monitoring, the patient was clearly at risk for undersedation, anxiety, and pain while paralyzed. The patient was also at risk for oversedation and prolonged ICU/ventilator days. The BIS facilitated withdrawal of NMB, weaning, extubation, and ICU discharge.

Case 14

A 57-year-old patient who had a history of HIV infection, PCP pneumonia, and progressive respiratory failure was intubated and received controlled ventilation to manage progressive hypoxemia and hypercapnia with clinical signs of severe respiratory distress. Initial therapy for pain/agitation consisted of lorazepam and fentanyl. Persistent ventilator dys-synchrony was managed initially by escalating lorazepam dosing and subsequently by NMB. During NMB, BIS monitoring was initiated and revealed a BIS value above 70, indicating potential risk for awareness and pain. In response, fentanyl was titrated upward accordingly, resulting in a decrease in BIS value to between 50 and 60. After 2 hours of increased opioid dosing, NMB was weaned off. Clinical assessment following recovery of neuromuscular function revealed a patient responsive to stimulation. Later that afternoon, the patient was localizing to a point in her abdomen indicating acute pain. Comprehensive abdominal assessment including CT scanning revealed an abdominal abscess, which was managed with percutaneous placement of a drainage catheter. The patient began weaning from ventilation the following day. EEG-based monitoring in this patient revealed a patient at risk for awareness and pain during NMB. In facilitating NMB withdrawal in response to optimal sedation and analgesia, evolving intra-abdominal pathology was revealed and successfully treated.

Case 15

A 66-year-old patient who had a history of bronchogenic lung cancer was admitted to the ICU to manage progressive respiratory failure. The patient's history included chronic pain for which he received oxycodone hydrochloride/acetaminophen, 2 tablets four times daily, before admission. Per his and his family's wishes, he consented to endotracheal intubation for management of severe respiratory failure. Sedation/analgesia was managed with lorazepam and morphine titrated to comfort and synchrony with ventilation. Progressive dys-synchrony with ventilation refractory to upward titration of lorazepam was managed with NMB. Approximately 2 hours following NMB, BIS monitoring was initiated and revealed that the patient was at risk for awareness and pain during NMB. Additional upward dose titration with morphine was initiated, which resulted in a decrease in the BIS value below 55. After determination of stable morphine and lorazepam dosing, NMB was weaned off and remained off, preserving the neurologic assessment and enabling clinical assessment of sedative/analgesic needs. EEG-based monitoring in this patient facilitated earlier withdrawal of NMB and identification of a patient at risk for awareness and pain while paralyzed. In addition, it identified a cerebral arousal response associated with attempted nasogastric intubation that raised the BIS value above 70, placing the patient at risk for breakthrough awareness and pain while paralyzed. Because of this information, the procedure was aborted and the BIS value quickly returned to baseline.

Within this sample of cases, BIS monitoring was decisive in 9 of 15 patients. Within this context, decisive is defined as (1) providing actionable, real-time information specific to care of a particular patient enabling or justifying a change in therapy, and (2) providing information that is not easily available by clinical examination of neurologic status or level of sedation. In 9 of 15 patients in this series, significant changes were made in therapy based on information obtained from EEG-based monitoring. In cases 2, 3, 10, 12, 14, and 15, the BIS facilitated withdrawal of NMB consequent to optimized sedation/analgesia. In these patients in whom earlier withdrawal of NMB was facilitated, cost avoidance was an advantage due to less use of these agents. Potential cost avoidance was an additional advantage in patient 3 and in patient 12 in whom weaning and extubation (subsequent to earlier withdrawal of NMB) was facilitated, with resulting avoidance of

additional ventilator and ICU days related to excessive sedation. In case 1, the BIS facilitated avoidance of NMB and enabled closer titration with propofol. In cases 9 and 11, the BIS enabled changes in sedative therapy during NMB.

Data analysis

Multiple paired observations (BIS and SAS) were obtained on 12 of 15 patients in this series. A total of 134 paired observations were obtained using the BIS A-2000; 52 with the BIS A-2000XP. The difference in observation totals between earlier and later versions of BIS technology places limits on generalizations that may be made from the available data. The SAS was regressed on the BIS A-2000 and then on the BIS A-2000XP. The author used a special clustering method to take the lack of independence of multiple pairs of observations (SAS, BIS) from the same patient into consideration in the linear regression analyses. Pearson correlations were presented. All statistical analyses were performed using Stata 7 (StataCorp LP, College Station, Texas). Regression analysis and Pearson correlations comparing the BIS A-2000 and the BIS A-2000XP versions are illustrated in Appendix 1.

A scatterplot of the SAS versus the BIS A-2000 shows a linear relationship (Fig. 1). For each unit increase in the BIS A-2000, on average, the SAS

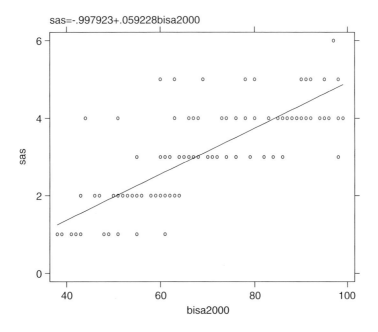

Fig. 1. A scatterplot of the SAS versus the BIS A-2000 showing a linear relationship.

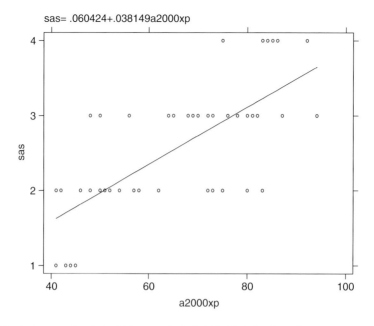

Fig. 2. A scatterplot of the SAS versus the BIS A-2000XP showing a linear relationship.

increases by 0.06 (95% confidence interval: 0.04–0.08, $P<0.001$). The corresponding correlation is $r=0.81$, $P<0.001$. In other words, the BIS A-2000 accounts for about 65% of the variation in the SAS. A scatterplot of the SAS versus the BIS A-2000XP shows a linear relationship (Fig. 2). For each unit increase in the BIS A-2000XP, the SAS increases by 0.04 (95% confidence interval: 0.02–0.06, $P=0.01$). The corresponding correlation is $r=0.73$. In other words, the BIS A-2000XP accounts for about 53% of the variation in the SAS.

Discussion

The data from this small case series of 15 patients represent a small sampling of patients for whom BIS monitoring may be effective and provide information that may be useful in determining direction of therapy. Data were collected on other patients as part of standard quality assurance activities and may be used, with limitations, as a basis for comparison with outcomes data obtained from patients monitored with the BIS adjunctively with clinical assessment. Within the data sample obtained by quality assurance activities (patients not monitored with the BIS) the following findings have significance. First is the incidence of awareness during NMB. One patient who had severe respiratory failure and was managed with NMB and lorazepam dosed at 10 mg/h experienced

awareness while paralyzed. On follow-up questioning, the patient reported the experience as a "bad dream" and accurately reported activities she experienced during that time. No patients who were monitored with the BIS reported incidence of awareness during NMB.

Four patients who were paralyzed to manage ventilator dys-synchrony also received varying doses of lorazepam by infusion. After achieving cardiopulmonary stability, NMB was weaned off and revealed deeply sedated patients who were unable to wean to extubation due to excessive sedation during NMB. These instances of oversedation contributed to additional ventilator days and ICU length of stay with concurrent risk of airway injury and ventilator-associated pneumonia. Based on the data from this case series, some conclusions may be drawn. One conclusion is that BIS monitoring may have a potential role in patients receiving NMB. In this subset of patients, BIS monitoring may identify patients at risk for oversedation, undersedation, and pain consequent to bedside procedures and may be used to guide therapy accordingly. A second conclusion is that the BIS may have a role in monitoring patients receiving deep sedation/analgesia to meet clinical goals such as ventilator management. A third conclusion is that because the clinical neurologic assessment is the gold standard for neurologic evaluation, clinical assessment will remain the gold standard for assessing level of sedation. In select circumstances such as NMB or deep sedation/analgesia in which the clinical assessment is compromised, equivocal, or otherwise unavailable, the BIS may have a role in monitoring and titration of sedative/hypnotic and analgesic therapy.

In 6 of 15 patients in this series, the BIS was not decisive but illustrated varying degrees of correlation with clinical assessment of sedation. In patients in whom clinical assessment of sedation remains reliable, clinical evaluation of sedation level should remain paramount. As such, if BIS monitoring adds no information beyond what is available by clinical assessment, it should generally not be used. In terms of correlation, the author found a moderately positive correlation between the BIS and clinical assessment of sedation. The BIS A-2000XP did not show improved correlation with clinical assessment of sedation in the patients in this series compared with the earlier version, the BIS A-2000. In both versions of BIS technology used, EMG activity remained a potential significant confounding factor in BIS determination and sedation assessment.

Summary

BIS monitoring is one example of additional technology used in the operating room setting by many anesthesia providers to guide drug therapy during surgical procedures. It was subsequently studied within the ICU environment. Potential benefits to BIS monitoring are illustrated from the data generated from this case series. Although studies illustrate varying degrees of correlation with clinical assessment tools for level of sedation, additional research is indicated to demonstrate specific benefits on clinical outcomes as measured by improved drug use, decreased ICU length of stay, and fewer ventilator days. The only potential risk associated with BIS monitoring is minor skin irritation in the area of sensor placement, which typically resolves following sensor removal. BIS values should be interpreted with caution due to the potential for EMG activity to cause an increase in BIS value independent of hypnotic state. BIS values should also always be interpreted within the context of the clinical examination and goals of therapy. Based on the data from this case series, additional implications cannot be made.

To optimize the BIS as a potential research tool, some recommendations can be made. First, being able to directly download historical data by the end user may markedly streamline data analysis and management and eliminate the need for large volumes of printouts to assess trends in BIS data. Second, data

downloads as currently provided from the BIS monitoring system consist of an Excel file (Microsoft) that has multiple columns of data variables and a separate Word file (Microsoft, Redmond, Washington) that contains event markers and times. Changing the format of data downloads to a single file, with the data corresponding to specific event markers that are highlighted, would greatly facilitate data management and analysis for the clinical researcher.

Acknowledgments

The author expresses utmost appreciation to the entire nursing staff in the Medical Intensive Care Unit at Albert Einstein Healthcare Network for their outstanding support, encouragement, and data collection efforts.

Appendix 1

Regression analysis and correlations between Sedation-Agitation Scale assessment and bispectral index monitoring using the BIS A-2000 or the BIS A-2000XP

BIS A-2000 and SAS: 134 paired observations: Pearson correlation

	BIS A-2000	SAS
BIS A-2000	1.0000	
SAS	0.8072	1.0000
	0.0000	

BIS A-2000 XP and SAS: 52 paired observations: Pearson correlation

	SAS	BIS A-2000XP
SAS	1.0000	
BIS A-2000XP	0.7271	1.0000
	0.0000	

Spearman correlation: BIS A-2000/SAS
    Number of observations=134
    Spearman ρ=0.8240
    Test of Ho: BIS A-2000 and SAS are independent
    Prob >|t|=0.0000

Spearman correlation: BIS A-2000XP/SAS
    Number of observations=52
    Spearman ρ=0.7348
    Test of Ho: BIS A-2000XP and SAS are independent
    Prob >|t|=0.0000

Regression analysis: BIS A-2000/SAS

Source	SS	df	MS
Number of observations	$=134$		
$F_{(1,132)}$	$=246.78$		
Model	25410.00	1	25410.00
Prob $>$ F	$=0.0000$		
Residual	13591.50	132	102.965909
R^2	$=0.6515$		
Adjusted R^2	$=0.6515$		
Total	39001.50	133	293.244361
Root MSE	$=10.147$		

Regression analysis: BIS A-2000XP/SAS.

Source	SS	df	MS
Number of observations	$=52$		
$F_{(1,50)}$	$=56.08$		
Model	6687.86068	1	6687.86068
Prob $>$ F	$=0.0000$		
Residual	5963.0624	50	119.261248
R^2	$=0.5286$		
Adjusted R^2	$=0.5192$		
Total	12650.9231	51	248.057315
Root MSE	$=10.921$		

References

[1] Bader MK, Arbour R, Sylvan P. Refractory increased intracranial pressure in severe traumatic brain injury: Barbiturate coma and bispectral index monitoring. AACN Clin Issues 2005;16(4):526–41.

[2] Arbour R. Continuous nervous system monitoring: EEG, the bispectral index and neuromuscular transmission. AACN Clin Issues 2003;14(2):185–207.

[3] Grissom TE, Grissom J. Neurologic monitoring in the ICU. Anesthesiology Online 2000. Available at: http://www.anesthesiologyonline.com/articles/onepage.cfm?chapter_id=34. Accessed December 19, 2001.

[4] Wallace BE, Wagner AK, Wagner EP, McDeavitt JT. A history and review of quantitative electroencephalography in traumatic brain injury. Head Trauma Rehabil 2001;16(2):165–90.

[5] Guerit JM. Medical technology assessment: EEG and evoked potentials in the intensive care unit. Neurophysiol Clin 1999;29:301–17.

[6] Rhoney DH, Parker D. Use of sedative and analgesic agents in neurotrauma patients: effects on cerebral physiology. Neurol Res 2001;23:237–59.

[7] Arbour R. Using bispectral index monitoring to detect potential breakthrough awareness and limit dura-

[8] Arbour R. Sedation and pain management in critically ill adults. Crit Care Nurs 2000;20(5):39–56.

[9] Rosow C, Manberg PJ. Bispectral index monitoring. Anesthiol Clin North America 1998;2:89–107.

[10] Huszar L. Clinical utility of evoked potentials. E-medicine 2001. Available at: http://www.emedicine.com/neuro/topic69.htm. Accessed February 19, 2001.

[11] Rampil IJ. A primer for EEG signal processing in anesthesia. Anesthesiology 1998;89:980–1002.

[12] Mascia MF, Koch M, Medicis JJ. Pharmacoeconomic impact of rational use guidelines on the provision of analgesia, sedation and neuromuscular blockade in critical care. Crit Care Med 2000;28(7):2300–6.

[13] De Johnge B, Bastuji-Garin S, Fangio P, et al. Sedation algorithm in critically ill patients without acute brain injury. Crit Care Med 2005;33(1):120–7.

[14] Kress JP, Pohlman AS, O'Connor MF, et al. Daily interruption of sedative infusions in critically ill patients undergoing mechanical ventilation. N Engl J Med 2000;342(20):1471–7.

[15] Jacobi J, Fraser GL, Coursin DB, et al. Clinical practice guidelines for the sustained use of sedatives and analgesics in the critically ill adult. Crit Care Med 2002;30(1):119–41.

[16] Riker RR, Fraser GL, Wilkins ML. Comparing the bispectral index and suppression ratio with burst suppression of the electroencephalogram during pentobarbital infusions in adult intensive care patients. Pharmacotherapy 2003;23:1087–93.

[17] Fabregas N, Gambus PL, Valero R, et al. Can bispectral index monitoring predict recovery of consciousness in patients with severe brain injury. Anesthesiology 2004;101(1):43–51.

[18] Vivien B, Di Maria S, Quattara A, et al. Overestimation of bispectral index in sedated intensive care unit patients revealed by administration of muscle relaxant. Anesthesiology 2003;99(1):9–17.

[19] Gill M, Haycock K, Green SM, et al. Can the bispectral index monitor the sedation of intubated ED adults. Am J Emerg Med 2004;22(2):76–82.

[20] Deogaonkar A, Gupta R, DeGeorgia M, et al. Bispectral index monitoring correlates with sedation scales in brain-injured patients. Crit Care Med 2004;32(12):2403–6.

[21] Kim DW, Kil HY, White PF. The effect of noise on the bispectral index during propofol sedation. Anesth Analg 2001;93:1170–3.

[22] Mondello E, Siliotti R, Noto G, et al. Bisoectral index in ICU: correlation with Ramsay Score on assessment of sedation level. J Clin Monit Comput 2002;17(5):271–7.

[23] Courtman SP, Wardburgh A, Petros AJ. Comparison of the bispectral index monitor with the Comfort score in assessing level of sedation of critically ill children. Intensive Care Med 2003;29:2239–46.

[24] Mourisse J, Booij L. Bispectral index detects period of cerebral hypoperfusion during cardiopulmo-

tion of neuromuscular blockade. Am J Crit Care 2004; 13(1):66–73.

nary bypass. J Cardiothorac Vasc Anesth 2003;17(1): 76–8.

[25] Azim N, Wang CY. Case report: the use of bispectral index during a cardiopulmonary arrest: a potential indicator of cerebral perfusion. Anesthesia 2004;59: 610–2.

[26] Vivien B, Langeron O, Riou B. Increase in bispectral index (BIS) while correcting a severe hypoglycemia. Anesth Analg 2002;95:824–5.

[27] Simmonds LE, Riker RR, Prato BS, et al. Assessing sedation during intensive care unit mechanical ventilation with the bispectral index and the sedation-agitation scale. Crit Care Med 1999;27(8):1499–504.

[28] Dasta JF, McLaughlin TP, Mody SH, et al. Daily cost of an intensive care unit day: the contribution of mechanical ventilation. Crit Care Med 2005;33(6): 1266–71.

ELSEVIER
SAUNDERS

Crit Care Nurs Clin N Am 18 (2006) 243–256

CRITICAL CARE
NURSING CLINICS
OF NORTH AMERICA

Recognizing and Treating Ischemic Insults to the Brain: The Role of Brain Tissue Oxygen Monitoring

Mary Kay Bader, RN, MSN, CCRN, CNRN

Mission Hospital, 27700 Medical Center Road, Mission Viejo, CA 92691, USA

Insults to the brain from trauma or subarachnoid hemorrhage (SAH) produce changes in structure, pressure dynamics, chemical balance, and blood flow. Ultimately, the delivery of oxygen to the cranial vault may become compromised. The devastating primary insult creates structural damage to neurons, vessels, and cranial nerves as well as compression of the brain and vasculature. The resulting edema and pathophysiologic processes further compromise the delivery of blood flow and oxygen to the brain. Patients who sustain severe traumatic brain injury (TBI) or SAH are vulnerable to secondary brain insults that can worsen their outcome [1–6]. Cerebral ischemia results from impaired autoregulation, systemic hypotension, hypoxia, hypocapnia, increased intracranial pressure (ICP), or vasospasm and leads to cerebral hypoxia [1–6] Andrews [7] stated "it is believed that the final common pathway in all acute brain injury is the failure of oxygen delivery (ischemia)." Detecting low oxygen states in the brain is vital to reducing secondary brain damage. Emerging technology, such as brain tissue oxygen monitoring by way of probes placed in the brain parenchyma, allows for the regional measurement of dissolved cerebral oxygen, and reflects the balance between oxygen delivery and consumption [1,4,6]. Use of this technology in the ICU assists practitioners in making decisions on interventions to reduce secondary brain injury. This article describes the potential application of the partial pressure of brain tissue oxygen ($PbtO_2$) monitoring technology in the care of patients who have sustained

TBI or SAH. To accomplish this objective, a review of the intracranial dynamics that are created by primary and secondary brain injury and the challenges of optimizing oxygen delivery to the injured brain are presented. Furthermore, interventions that facilitate cerebral oxygen supply and reduce oxygen consumption are identified. Finally, application of this technology is highlighted by using case vignettes of patients who have experienced TBI or SAH.

The brain under assault: impact of traumatic brain injury and subarachnoid hemorrhage

Severe TBI and SAH are different mechanisms that produce similar pathophysiologic changes that can lead to neuronal injury and death. To understand how each impacts the brain, a brief overview of their pathophysiology is presented.

Traumatic brain injury: the dynamics of primary and secondary injury

In TBI, a mechanism produces a primary injury to the cranial vault. This primary injury occurs at the time of the event and the damage caused cannot be altered [2,8]. There is structural damage to the neurons and disruption in neurochemical processes [9]. Various types of injuries are produced, including shearing of the neurons and injury to the vessels of the brain [8]. These insults result in hemorrhages, brain tissue edema, and compression of the brain and its structures [8]. Because the brain and its contents, including blood and cerebrospinal fluid (CSF), normally occupy and share space inside the cranial

E-mail address: badermk@aol.com

vault in a 80%:10%:10% balance, an increase in one of the three must lead to a decrease in the other two (Monro-Kellie doctrine). When the capacity for the brain contents to accommodate for increases in the volume is exhausted, any further increases lead to a dramatic increase in pressure. Therefore, the primary injuries of hemorrhage and edema can lead to increasing ICP and secondary injury by reducing blood flow delivery to the cranial vault.

Following the primary injury, additional processes produce secondary insult to the brain [2]. This type of injury occurs at a cellular level and has many causes [2]. Chesnut [8] divided these two processes into those that arise from the traumatic event or changes to the brain and vasculature that occur following the primary insult, and those that are caused by extracerebral events.

The processes that arise from the initial injury include development of cerebral edema, alteration of cerebral blood flow (CBF) and metabolic rate, impaired autoregulation, and chemical derangements [8,9]. Cerebral edema is a direct result of damage to neurons and the disruption of membrane stability, cytoskeletal function, and axon transport mechanisms that lead to axonal swelling [9]. The edema can lead to an increase in the tissue volume in the cranial vault. If significant, it can produce mass effect and increase ICP.

Following TBI, there is an alteration in CBF or cerebral metabolic rate of oxygen [10]. Martin and colleagues' [11] study on CBF after TBI revealed three distinct patterns of flow. First, there is a state of hypoperfusion and a decrease in CBF in the first 24 hours after injury (day 0). Earlier studies confirm this finding [12,13]. The cause of the decrease in CBF may be an increase in distal microcirculatory resistance as well as intravascular clot formation [10,11]. After the first 24 hours, CBF increases. This occurs from days 1 through 5 and exceeds the cerebral metabolic demand for oxygen [11]. This phenomenon could lead to impairment in metabolic coupling that cause vascular engorgement, swelling, and increased ICP [14]. In the third phase, CBF is altered beginning somewhere on days 4 or 5 and continues through day 14. This phase is characterized by slow flow from vasospasm. Autoregulation is another important factor that alters CBF. Pressure autoregulation is the ability of the brain to maintain a constant CBF in the face of changing blood pressure (BP) or cerebral perfusion pressure (CPP) [15]. In patients who have sustained TBI, CPP is measured when an ICP monitor is placed. CPP is equal to the mean arterial pressure (MAP) minus the ICP. Optimal CPP levels differ in patients, probably as a result of whether pressure autoregulation is intact or impaired. The impairment of autoregulation can contribute to cerebral ischemia, and thus, reduced CBF and oxygen delivery [5,15].

Cerebral metabolism is altered severely by the loss or decrease in blood flow that shifts the metabolism of oxygen from aerobic to anaerobic [9]. It also is impacted by depressed cerebral activity, inflammatory response, mitochondrial dysfunction, and the uncoupling of autoregulation [2,9,10]. Finally, chemical derangements, including calcium-induced cellular damage, glutamate excitotoxicity, and free radical formation, lead to cell damage and death [9]. Research continues in an effort to understand these intense cellular and chemical derangements and to find drugs that might ameliorate the changes.

Extracerebral causes of secondary brain injury include hypoxia, hypotension, hypocapnia, impaired autoregulation, acidosis, and hyperglycemia [1,2,4,5, 8,16,17]. Each factor produces a reduction in oxygen delivery or blood flow (hypoxia, hypotension, hypocapnia, or anemia) or an alteration in neurochemical processes (acidosis and hyperglycemia). Appreciation of each of these factors is imperative for the reduction of secondary brain injury.

The two most commonly linked causes, hypoxia and hypotension, are seen in patients who have sustained TBI. This is especially true in the presence of multisystem trauma. In numerous studies hypoxia was identified as increasing the morbidity and mortality of patients who had a severe TBI [18–21]. Gracias and colleagues' [16] pilot study used brain tissue oxygen measurements and reported that episodes of cerebral hypoxia—defined as a partial pressure of brain tissue oxygen ($PbtO_2$) of less than 20 mm Hg—are associated with a significantly lower mean PaO_2. Two recent studies that examined hypoxia and hypotension in severe TBI found that hypotension was associated significantly with worsening outcomes, whereas hypoxia did not impact mortality significantly [22,23]. Strong evidence in the literature demonstrates that one or more episodes of hypotension experienced in the prehospital or in-hospital setting correlated with increased morbidity and mortality [2,18,19,21–25].

Hypocapnia, a reduction of the $PaCO_2$, causes vasoconstriction of cerebral blood vessels and leads to a reduction in CBF [26]. This reduction decreases oxygen delivery to the brain, as represented by decreases in $PbtO_2$, and may produce cerebral ischemia [1,27–29].

Acidosis was identified as a secondary brain injury factor in Jeremitsky and colleagues' [2] study. They found that a base deficit of greater than −4 correlated with a longer stay in the ICU. Mulvey and colleagues [9] reported than an increase in lactate concentration and low tissue pH correlated with poor outcome in animal and human studies. Hyperglycemia—blood glucose levels greater than 200 mg/dL—correlated with an increase in worst neurologic outcomes [30–32]. Jeremitsky and colleagues [2] found that hyperglycemia was associated with increased mortality and longer hospital stays. The exact mechanism may be related to an increase in production of lactate, which creates neuronal injury [30].

Aneurysmal subarachnoid hemorrhage

Aneurysmal SAH carries a high mortality and morbidity because of devastating primary and secondary insults. The primary hemorrhage—from blood rapidly escaping a ruptured aneurysm into the subarachnoid space, brain parenchyma, or ventricles—creates compression of structures and increased ICP. Secondary insults can occur, including impaired autoregulation, hypotension, hypoxia, hydrocephalus, cardiac complications, hypovolemia, vasospasm, and increased metabolism from seizures and pyrexia [6,33,34]. Impaired autoregulation, hypotension, and hypoxia were alluded to in the previous section. Hydrocephalus—a build-up of CSF in the ventricles—causes increased ICP because of an increase in CSF volume. Cardiac complications and hypovolemia may impair the delivery of blood to the brain, which leads to inadequate delivery of oxygen. Vasospasm—arterial narrowing of the proximal intracranial vessels—may occur in 60% to 70% of all patients who have an aneurysmal SAH [3]. Thirty percent will suffer a delayed ischemic neurologic deficit from the reduction in CBF to the vascular territory [3]. Lastly, seizures and fever increase the use of oxygen by the brain and should be avoided to prevent further injury [33].

Significant factors contribute to secondary brain injury in severe TBI and SAH. Detecting these events requires intense vigilance by practitioners. Traditionally, hemodynamic and ICP monitors are used as a primary means to guide therapies to keep brain pressure within normal limits and to optimize CPP. These monitors are limited in their ability to detect changes in cerebral oxygenation or blood flow. New technologies are emerging in the ICU setting to monitor other variables. One of the technologies, brain tissue oxygen monitoring, has undergone intense study and is being used in many neuro-ICU centers in Europe and the United States. The advantages of monitoring brain oxygen tension continuously are that it brings practitioners closer to identifying ischemic episodes

and ensures adequate oxygen delivery to the injured brain through various interventions.

Monitoring brain tissue oxygen

The measurement of $PbtO_2$ is accomplished by placing a small, oxygen-sensitive probe into the brain tissue. Measuring $PbtO_2$ in this manner reflects local or regional oxygen tension. Debate exists over whether to place the specific catheter on the injured side of the brain or in the contralateral side of the brain. Haitsma and Maas [35] suggested that placing the catheter near the injury reflects local brain oxygen levels, whereas placing it in the normal or undamaged brain reflects global cerebral oxygenation (Fig. 1). In patients who have an aneurysmal SAH, the catheter's most desirable placement is in the arterial zone of probable vasospasm. The resulting measurements of $PbtO_2$ are reflective of the balance between the supply of oxygen and the demand for oxygen in the brain tissue [35].

Types of brain tissue oxygen monitors

Two brain oxygen monitoring systems are available commercially. The origin of both systems is a Clark-type electrode that measures oxygen tension polarographically in blood or tissue [35].

The Paratrend system (Diametrics Medical, High Wycombe, U.K.) originally was designed to be used in the intravascular measurement of oxygen, carbon dioxide, pH, and temperature [36]. Three sensors were placed over a 4-cm long probe that was 0.5 mm in diameter. The Paratrend system was altered in 1999 to incorporate fluorescent technology, but its measuring length was shortened to 2 cm [36]. The new catheter was called the Neurotrend (Codman, Raynam, Massachusetts). The oxygen-sensing section of the probe was reduced to 1.4 mm. Because of the limited area of oxygen sensing, there seemed to be more variability in the $PbtO_2$ measurements compared with the other systems with larger monitoring area [36].

The LICOX brain oxygen monitoring system (Integra Neurosciences, Plainsboro, New Jersey) uses the Clark electrode, which is 0.5 mm in diameter and has a 5-mm long oxygen-sensing area [35,37]. The original LICOX system has two separate small probes (0.8 mm in size) that are placed down separate channels into an introducer (Fig. 2A) [37]. The oxygen and temperature probes are passed approximately 25 to 35 mm into the white matter of the brain, usually in the frontal lobe (see Fig. 1).

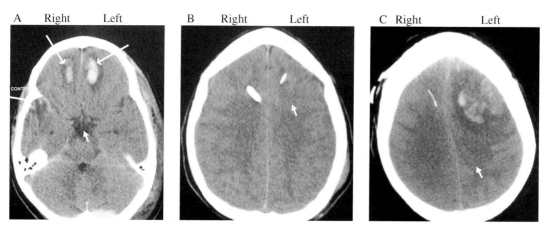

Fig. 1. Placement of the brain tissue oxygen probe in the brain. (*A*) CT scan of brain with left and right frontal contusions, with left contusions larger than right. (*B*) CT scan of brain of same patient demonstrating placement of the brain oxygen catheter on the left (predominant side of injury), which is indicative of local or regional oxygen. Note the ICP catheter in the right hemisphere. (*C*) CT scan of brain with left stroke and hemorrhage present and brain oxygen catheter in right hemisphere. This reflects the placement of the catheter in the noninjured side, which is more reflective of a global oxygen picture.

The catheters measure oxygen and brain temperature separately. The oxygen measurement requires temperature to give accurate $PbtO_2$ levels. In the past year, the LICOX catheter has been altered; the oxygen and temperature sensors have been placed on one catheter (Fig. 2B). The PMO catheter has a sampling surface area of 18 mm^2 with an oxygen-sensing length of 7 mm [38]. The temperature sensing area is 4.5 mm in length. The PMO catheter has a slightly larger diameter (0.65 mm). The overall length of the catheter is 460 mm. This catheter can be placed through a bolt system or tunneled into the parenchyma, which is especially useful in infants and toddlers with thin skulls. Once in place, the catheter(s) requires a "settling in" period from 10 to 120 minutes because of potential local tissue trauma during placement [37].

The oxygen probe must be placed in "viable tissue," not in contused or infarcted brain. The position of the catheter should be assessed by CT of the brain [35]. A catheter response test can be performed by increasing the fraction of inspired oxygen (FIO_2) to 100% for 2 minutes. Appropriately placed catheters respond with a significant increase in the $PbtO_2$ while the FIO_2 is increased [35].

Several studies have been undertaken to determine the safety and reliability of the oxygen probes/systems. Nine studies demonstrated no infectious complications [1,17,29,39–44]. A study by Dings and colleagues [43] reported two small intraparenchymal hematomas in 118 patients. Clinical experience at Mission Hospital, with 200 catheters placed in the

last 4 years, produced no infections and two small hematomas around the catheter site.

Measured values of partial pressure of brain tissue oxygen

After the catheters are placed and verified to be in correct position, the measurements (in mm Hg) will be displayed. Because of the different oxygen-sensing areas on the two different systems, studies found different ranges of normal and abnormal [35,36]. In an attempt to test the two different probes in a zero-oxygen solution, Valadka and colleagues [45] found that the Paratrend probes gave an average reading of 7.0 mm Hg compared with 0.3 mm Hg for the LICOX probes. The investigators stated the Paratrend "overestimated PO_2 when values were near zero." The Paratrend/Neurotrend catheter has been examined in a limited number of human studies. Nemani and Manley [36] cited ethical constraints as limiting the pursuit of validating "normal brain oxygen levels" in noninjured humans. One study of patients who underwent neurosurgery revealed a normal average of 37 mm Hg in patients with intact circulation in noncompromised brain and an average of 10 mm Hg in regions with compromised circulation [46]. Zauner and colleagues [47] studied patients who had sustained head injuries. The average $PbtO_2$ was 39 mm Hg in patients who had a good outcome, whereas patients whose levels were less than 31 mm Hg sustained moderate to severe dis-

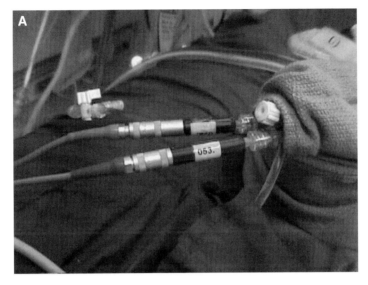

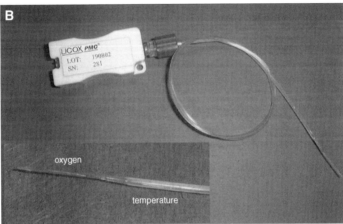

Fig. 2. (*A*) Original LICOX catheter probes with oxygen (blue) and temperature (green) cables that connect to probes that are inserted into the brain of a patient who has a severe TBI. (*B*) The PMO LICOX catheter. Inset: oxygen and temperature sensors are on one catheter. (Fig. 2B courtesy of Integra Neurosciences; with permission.)

ability. Patients who died or were in a persistent vegetative state had an average value of 19 mm Hg [47]. Doppenberg and colleagues [48] studied 25 patients who had a severe TBI; 4 patients with $PbtO_2$ values of less than 18 mm Hg died.

Using the LICOX system, Maas and colleagues [49] found $PbtO_2$ levels of 25 to 30 mm Hg in un-injured white matter of frontal lobes. Sarrafzadeh and colleagues [44] determined that uninjured areas of brain tissue had $PbtO_2$ values of 20 to 35 mm Hg. Meixensberger and colleagues [50] placed surface probes in normal brain of patients who underwent craniotomy, and reported a mean $PbtO_2$ of 47.9 mm Hg. Because of the lack of studies in normal brains, it has been difficult to identify true normal values.

Hlatky and colleagues [51] estimated normal values of $PbtO_2$ to be between 20 and 40 mm Hg. This range gave a target $PbtO_2$ with the understanding that true "normals" have not been validated and that various intracranial pathologies may cause different CBF and oxygen states.

Several studies have provided insight into "critical" or abnormal levels of $PbtO_2$ using the LICOX monitor. van den Brink and colleagues [17] studied 101 comatose patients who had TBIs and found that the duration of time and depth of local tissue hypoxia correlated with outcomes at 6 months. The survivors had significantly higher $PbtO_2$ levels during the monitoring period than did the patients who died. Lower $PbtO_2$ levels were related to a greater risk for death [17]. The investigators found that a $PbtO_2$ of less than 15 mm Hg for longer than 30 minutes or less than 10 mm Hg for 10 minutes correlated with a statistically significant risk for death. In one study of 39 patients, the investigators found that a $PbtO_2$ of less than 15 mm Hg correlated with a greater chance of death. A value of less than 6 mm Hg at any time was associated with a greater risk for dying [45]. In a study 35 patients who had TBI, Bardt and colleagues [52] found that episodes of a $PbtO_2$ of less than 10 mm Hg for more than 30 minutes correlated with a poor neurologic outcome; this occurred in 23 of the patients. At 6 months 55.6% had died, 22.2% were severely disabled or in a persistent vegetative state, and 22.2% had a favorable outcome. van Santbrink and colleagues [41] studied 22 patients who had TBI, and reported that 4 of 5 patients with a $PbtO_2$ of less than 5 mm Hg died. The only survivor had a cerebral contusion in the location of the probe, which may have confounded the accuracy of the readings. Palmer and Bader [53] reported that 11 of 72 patients who had varying neurologic diagnoses and LICOX catheters in place experienced brain death. All 11 patients had their $PbtO_2$ decrease to 0 mm Hg, whereas none of the remaining patients 61 had $PbtO_2$ levels of 0 mm Hg.

It is apparent that the type of oxygen system that is used to measure $PbtO_2$ impacts the range of normal and abnormal levels. Although more research is needed to validate "normal" $PbtO_2$ levels, most practitioners recognize that lower levels of $PbtO_2$ tend to correlate with poorer neurologic outcomes. It is prudent to consider the $PbtO_2$ value in relation to pulmonary/cerebrovascular physiology, as well as pulmonary, hemodynamic, and cerebral variables. Practitioners must be knowledgeable in both of these areas.

Pulmonary/cerebrovascular physiology

Fundamental to understanding the use of $PbtO_2$ monitoring is the team's ability to relate concepts of systemic oxygenation to oxygen delivery to the brain. The functions of the lungs are to ventilate the alveoli, diffuse gases into and out of blood, and bring blood flow to the lungs to transport blood rich in oxygen (O_2) and low in carbon dioxide (CO_2) to the body [54]. O_2 is transported in the blood bound to hemoglobin (SaO_2) or dissolved in the plasma of arterial blood (PaO_2). Approximately 20 mL of O_2 is carried per 100 mL of blood; most O_2 is carried by hemoglobin but a small amount is dissolved in plasma. Less hemoglobin in the blood results in a lower oxygen-carrying capacity. O_2 quickly binds to hemoglobin as it crosses from the lungs to the vasculature. It stays bound until it is released at the tissue level. The oxyhemoglobin curve is an S-shaped curve, which illustrates the concepts of the relationship between PO_2 and SaO_2. Varying clinical situations impact the affinity of O_2 to stay bound to hemoglobin versus oxygen's ability to dissociate from hemoglobin at the tissue level. A right shift correlates with hemoglobin giving up its bound O_2 to the tissues. Acidosis, high CO_2, increased temperature, and high levels of 2-3 diphosphoglycerate (DPG) tend to increase the dissociation of O_2 from hemoglobin [54]. A shift to the left correlates with the affinity for O_2 to stay bound to hemoglobin instead of unloading at the tissue level. Alkalosis, hypocapnia, decreased temperature, and low levels of 2-3 DPG tend to decrease the release of O_2 to the tissues [54]. The delivery of O_2 to the tissues of the brain is dependent on the vasculature.

The cerebrovasculature must deliver the O_2 and other nutrients to the brain on a continuous basis. Approximately 15% of the cardiac output is directed to the brain [36]. Generally, when practitioners describe oxygen delivery to the body, the cardiac output is used as a major factor in calculating the delivery. When describing oxygen delivery to the brain, CBF must be factored into the equation. CBF is the CPP divided by the cerebrovascular resistance. CBF is influenced by influx/efflux pressure, vascular radius, and blood viscosity [56]. CPP, pressure autoregulation, flow–metabolism coupling, and metabolic chemicals impact CBF [56]. CPP and pressure autoregulation were alluded to in a previous section. Flow–metabolism coupling reflects the concept that CBF changes to meet the demand for oxygen or metabolism. Therefore, as cerebral metabolism increases, CBF increases. Conversely, as cerebral metabolism decreases, CBF decreases [56]. The metabolic impact on CBF is related to changes in PaO_2, $PaCO_2$, and acid–base balance. Vasoconstriction occurs at hyperbaric levels of PaO_2 and decreased levels of $PaCO_2$ [56]. Johnston and colleagues [57] noted that the ability of the cerebral vessels to constrict to high PaO_2 probably is limited. CBF is more responsive to changes in $PaCO_2$ than PaO_2 [57]. For every 1 mm Hg decrease in $PaCO_2$, there is a 2% to 3% reduction in CBF between $PaCO_2$ levels of 20 and 80 mm Hg. The reverse principle holds true for increases in $PaCO_2$ [56]. When PaO_2 is less than 60 mm Hg, the cerebral vessels vasodilate [57]. PaO_2 levels of 25 mm Hg double the CBF [57]. The pH of the blood impacts CBF; acidosis causes vasodilatation and alkalosis causes vasoconstriction [56]. All of these factors play an integral part in the delivery of oxygenated blood to the brain. After blood is delivered, oxygen normally is consumed in higher amounts than in other living tissues.

The brain consumes 30% to 40% of the oxygen that is delivered [55]. The consumption of O_2 is increased in the presence of severe TBI and with the release of neuroexcitatory chemicals from damaged neurons. It also occurs in hyperthermia and seizures [56].

Adequate oxygenation of the brain is a balance between oxygen supply, oxygen delivery, and oxygen consumption. Measuring oxygen directly in the brain tissue brings practitioners closer to assessing oxygen content and delivery [17]. In addition, it reflects a parameter that is capable of evaluating pulmonary, hemodynamic, and cerebral variables to detect events that lead to oxygen deficits and cerebral ischemia.

Impact of pulmonary, hemodynamic, and cerebral variables on partial pressure of brain tissue oxygen

Research has examined the impact of pulmonary, hemodynamic, and cerebral variables on $PbtO_2$ responses. Interventions that are directed at manipulating these variables, and their impact on $PbtO_2$, have been reported in the literature. Translating the outcomes of the research findings and applying them to a patient requires an understanding of the underlying physiology and a coordinated team effort. Specific interventions to increase $PbtO_2$ may impact other systems. The team must be practicing "on the same page" as it strives to maintain adequate cerebral oxygenation while diminishing potential harm to other areas.

Pulmonary variables, events, and interventions

Titrating FIO_2 and $PaCO_2$ have been investigated in several studies that explored the impact on $PbtO_2$. van Santbrink and colleagues' [41] study of 22 patients who had sustained TBI found that patients who were preoxygenated with 100% FIO_2 (hyperoxia) before suctioning had increases in their $PbtO_2$. Decreasing $PaCO_2$ (hyperventilation) decreased $PbtO_2$ [41]. van den Brink and colleagues [29] studied 82 patients who had TBI and noted changes in $PbtO_2$ with various interventions. In a subgroup of 7 patients, the lack of preoxygenation with 100% FIO_2 before suctioning led to decreases in $PbtO_2$. In 142 suctioning episodes in which FIO_2 was increased to 100% 5 minutes before suction, the $PbtO_2$ increased. Gopinath and colleagues [58] investigated

two types of oxygen monitoring systems and the impact episodes of hyperoxia and hyperventilation. The $PbtO_2$ was impacted greatly with increases in $PbtO_2$ during hyperoxia, whereas hyperventilation caused decreases in $PbtO_2$. Menzel and colleagues [59] increased the FIO_2 to 100% for 6 hours, and discovered that the $PbtO_2$ increased and improved O_2 supply to the brain. Tolias and colleagues [60] studied 52 patients who had TBI and were given 100% FIO_2 for the first 24 hours after admission, and compared them with a control group in whom FIO_2 was not increased to 100%. They noted that the hyperoxia treatment increased the $PbtO_2$ levels by an average of 36 mm Hg during the 100% FIO_2. In addition to studying $PbtO_2$, they measured brain chemicals. In the microdialysis brain fluid, the group that received treatment had reduced glutamate, lactate, lactate/glucose ratios, and lactate/pyruvate ratios that were indicative of improved brain oxidation metabolism. When compared with the control group, the hyperoxia-treated group had significant reductions in ICP during and after the treatment. Reinert and colleagues' [61] study of 20 patients found similar results, with $PbtO_2$ increasing after hyperoxia. Likewise, the brain microdialysis lactate had decreased. Another study of 8 patients who had TBI revealed similar findings between FIO_2, $PbtO_2$, and lactate, except that the other microdialysis substrates did not change [62]. Studies that explored the impact of hyperventilation on $PbtO_2$ found decreases in $PbtO_2$ with corresponding decreases in $PaCO_2$ [1,27,28,63,64].

Critical neurosurgical patients unable to protect their airway because of a decrease in their level of consciousness are intubated with an endotracheal tube and maintained on a ventilator. Support of the airway usually is accomplished by monitoring PaO_2 and $PaCO_2$ as well as ventilatory parameters. Many investigators maintain that a PaO_2 of 100 mm Hg is adequate, but one must consider that it may or may not ensure adequate $PbtO_2$. The dangers of hypoxia and hypocapnia were alluded to in previous sections on major causes of secondary brain injury. Hyperventilation, once the mainstay of treatment for TBI, has been shown to worsen neurologic outcomes. Studies cited above confirm the impact of decreasing $PaCO_2$ on $PbtO_2$. In patients who have an aneurysmal SAH and who are at risk for cerebral vasoconstriction from vasospasm, decreasing $PaCO_2$ to less than 35 mm Hg may be harmful. Caution must be exercised when titrating $PaCO_2$ in the patient who has a brain injury.

Determining the optimal PaO_2 and $PaCO_2$ is accomplished by observing the $PbtO_2$ response and should be balanced with the condition of the lungs. Continuous monitoring of CO_2 by way of end-tidal capnography is helpful to detect changes that may be harmful to the brain.

Often, patients who have a severe TBI or SAH experience pneumonia as a consequence of their injury and ventilatory management. Some may progress to acute respiratory distress syndrome (ARDS). One study examined using prone positioning in patients who had SAH and ARDS. They found that PaO_2 and $PbtO_2$ increased significantly when patients were turned from supine to prone. Although the researchers found that the CPP decreased, mainly from an increase in ICP during the proning, the $PbtO_2$ improved despite these changes [65].

The oxygen-carrying capacity of hemoglobin and its influence on $PbtO_2$ were studied by Smith and colleagues [66]. In 35 patients who required packed red blood cell transfusions, the $PbtO_2$ increased after the transfusion in 26 patients (CPP and ICP were unchanged before, during, and after the transfusions), and decreased in 9 patients. The age of the transfused blood was 19 ± 10 days and 24 ± 10 days, respectively.

Applying the concepts that are related to pulmonary variables in patients who have TBI or SAH takes communication between disciplines and critical thinking. The following vignettes present the impact that the pulmonary system has on $PbtO_2$.

Vignette 1: traumatic brain injury

TH, an 18-year-old man, sustained a head injury, pulmonary contusions, bilateral pneumothoraces, lacerated liver, and ruptured spleen in a high-speed, rollover car accident. After initial resuscitation in the Emergency Department (ED), an ICP monitor, LICOX monitor, and three chests tubes were placed in the operating room. He also underwent an exploratory laparotomy for repair of his liver and spleen. Because surgeons were unable to close his abdomen, prolene mesh was applied and covered with a black sponge that was cut to fit the wound. A wound Vac was placed and suction was applied. Orders were given to titrate the $PaCO_2$ and FIO_2 to keep the ICP at less than 20 mm Hg and the $PbtO_2$ at greater than 20 mm Hg. On day 3, the $PbtO_2$ decreased suddenly from 21 mm Hg to 12 mm Hg. At the time the ICP was 14 mm Hg and the CPP was 72 mm Hg. An immediate arterial blood gas level was obtained on a FIO_2 of 50%, which revealed an acute decrease in his PaO_2. The PaO_2 had decreased from 180 mm Hg to 71 mm Hg. The $PaCO_2$ went from 35 mm Hg to 44 mm Hg. The respiratory care practitioner increased the FIO_2 to 100%. Despite increasing the FIO_2, the $PbtO_2$ hovered around 14 mm Hg. The intensivist performed an emergent bronchoscopy, which showed multiple mucous plugs in the right lung. After the bronchoscopy, the $PbtO_2$ increased to 38 mm Hg. The FIO_2 was weaned down from 100% to 50% over the next hour. The FIO_2 was reduced to 50% and the $PbtO_2$ stabilized at 25 mm Hg.

Vignette 2: aneurysm

CA, a 40-year-old man, ruptured a giant cerebral aneurysm on his left anterior cerebral artery. His history included hypertension and a two pack per day smoking habit. He was in a coma and extensor posturing on arrival to the ED. After intubation and lines were placed, CA underwent an emergent cerebral angiogram. Three meters of coils were threaded into the giant aneurysm to occlude it. After the coiling procedure, an ICP, LICOX, and pulmonary artery catheter were placed. CA was admitted to the Neurology ICU. On day 4 when the day shift began, CA's $PbtO_2$ was 45 mm Hg, his ICP was 19 mm Hg, his systolic BP was 140 mm Hg, and his O_2 saturation was 100%. He was on 45% FIO_2 with a PaO_2 of 120 mm Hg and a $PaCO_2$2 of 35 mm Hg. Five hours into the shift he developed pulmonary issues. CA's $PbtO_2$ decreased to 15 mm Hg and his ICP hovered in the low twenties. His FIO_2 was increased to 100% with little change to the $PbtO_2$. After checking the chest radiograph, the intensivist performed a bronchoscopy, which revealed a large mucous plug. Believing that the patient would do better on a different ventilator mode, changes were made to the ventilator settings. The positive end-expiratory pressure (PEEP) was increased from 8 mm Hg to 12 mm Hg, the tidal volumes were decreased from 750 mL to 450 mL, and the rate was increased from 14 to 22 breaths per minute. This change improved his PaO_2 to 320 mm Hg, but increased the $PaCO_2$ from 35 mm Hg to 44 mm Hg. The impact to the cranial vault was dramatic. CA's ICP increased to 56 mm Hg and his $PbtO_2$ decreased to 3 mm Hg. After an emergent scan of his brain revealed no intracranial changes, a discussion was held among the team. The different ventilator strategy had increased his PaO_2 but had produced astounding changes to his ICP and $PbtO_2$. A decision was made to reprogram the ventilator by decreasing the PEEP and rate while increasing the tidal volumes back to 750 mL. The team watched the end tidal CO_2 decrease by 9 mm Hg. Within 1 minute, the ICP decreased to 15 mm Hg and the $PbtO_2$ increased to 48 mm Hg. The FIO_2 was weaned back to 50% and CA's $PbtO_2$ settled at 35 mm Hg.

In both cases, the lungs and ventilator parameters had an astounding impact on the $PbtO_2$. The $PbtO_2$ changed before any other parameters.

Hemodynamic variables, events, and interventions

Maintaining an adequate CPP promotes delivery of blood to the brain. When CPP is inadequate, ICP increases and $PbtO_2$ may decrease. It is believed that when autoregulation is intact, CBF does not change between CPPs of 60 mm Hg to 140 mm Hg [67]. When CPP decreases to less than a threshold of approximately 60 mm Hg, there is a potential for a decrease in CBF and the development of cerebral ischemia. When autoregulation is impaired, the brain becomes dependent on the MAP/CPP for adequate blood flow and oxygen delivery. As ICP increases, the CPP may decrease unless the MAP is increased. Vespa's [67] review of several studies—in the search for an optimal CPP threshold in patients who have TBI—found that no correct or optimal CPP threshold can be applied to all patients. He concluded that different areas of the brain may require different CPP levels, and that the CPP threshold may change from day to day. The selection of an adequate CPP must be individualized to each patient. Incorporating other cerebral measures, such as ICP, $PbtO_2$, jugular venous oximetry, and microdialysis, might assist practitioners in determining the optimal CPP threshold for the patient.

Three early studies on optimal CPP thresholds found that when CPP was less than 60 mm Hg, $PbtO_2$ decreased [29,39,63]. One of the studies noted that when changing intravenous tubing of vasopressors, the CPP decreased significantly and led to dramatic decreases in the $PbtO_2$ of 4 patients [29]. Reinert and colleagues' [61] study on the effects of increasing CPP on $PbtO_2$ noted that $PbtO_2$ increased as CPP was increased, up to a CPP level of 78 mm Hg. After that point, further elevations of CPP did not increase the $PbtO_2$. Meixensberger and colleagues' [4] study on $PbtO_2$-guided therapy in patients who had TBI compared two groups of patients. Forty patients were cared for by managing the ICP/CPP only, whereas 53 patients were managed using ICP-, CPP-, and $PbtO_2$-targeted parameters. The investigators noted that there were several episodes of low $PbtO_2$ when CPP was decreased. Increasing the CPP resulted in increases in the $PbtO_2$. There was not a statistical difference in the outcome between the two groups at 6 months, although there was a positive trend in the latter group. Stochetti and colleagues [68] cautioned that despite normal CPP values in their study of 9 patients, there were episodes of low $PbtO_2$ values. They found that increasing the CPP to higher levels than normal increased the $PbtO_2$ [68]. In a study on patients who had aneurysms, investigators found a correlation between MAP and $PbtO_2$. When MAP was decreased to less than 80 mm Hg there was a progressive decrease in the $PbtO_2$ levels [6]. Johnston and colleagues [69] pointed out that below the autoregulatory threshold of optimal CPP, the $PbtO_2$ was dependent on CPP. Increased $PbtO_2$ resulted from increases in CPP. Determining the correct CPP threshold for patients who had TBI or SAH was studied by Soehle and colleagues [5]. They found that increasing CPP did not increase $PbtO_2$ when autoregulation was intact. When autoregulation was impaired, increasing CPP caused the $PbtO_2$ to increase. The researchers also described a phenomenon whereby increasing CPP caused the $PbtO_2$ to decrease in a patient who had intact autoregulation. They called this an inverse $PbtO_2$-autoregulation state.

Enhancing the CPP to just above the threshold was shown to be beneficial in patients, recognizing that thresholds will differ between patients. When autoregulation is intact, increasing CPP to greater than 60 mm Hg may not be necessary. If autoregulation is impaired, the optimal CPP threshold needs to be determined based on $PbtO_2$ and ICP response. To enhance CPP, intravenous fluids are used to ensure euvolemia. Vasopressors are used if further enhancement of CPP is needed once volume loaded.

Vasospasm in patients who have SAH results in vasoconstriction of blood vessels and a decrease in oxygen delivery. One study assessed whether $PbtO_2$ decreased when vasospasm occurred. There were transient decreases in $PbtO_2$ with vasospasm in 7 patients who had SAH but the levels never decreased to less than 20 mm Hg [70]. A case study reported a decrease in the $PbtO_2$ to 2 mm Hg with corresponding angiographic confirmation of 80% stenosis of the left internal carotid artery (ICA). After angioplasty, the $PbtO_2$ increased from 1.5 mm Hg to 40 mm Hg [71]. Patients who have aneurysmal SAH receive nimodipine to mediate vasospasm. The impact of nimodipine administration on $PbtO_2$ was studied in 11 patients with SAH. The investigators found that the $PbtO_2$ decreased significantly in 7 of 11 patients, and it persisted for up to 2 hours [72].

Vasospasm has the potential to impact oxygen delivery to the brain. Optimal management includes volume loading and MAP enhancement with vasopressors Observing for a potential decline in the $PbtO_2$ may help to identify episodes of ischemia in these patients.

Vignette 3: aneurysm revisited

CA, described in vignette 2, had a precipitous decline in his $PbtO_2$ on day 10 after his SAH. His $PbtO_2$ decreased from 24 mm Hg to 16 mm Hg. A transcranial doppler exam was obtained which demonstrated an increase in velocities in the right anterior cerebral artery (ACA) distribution. CA was taken to the angiogram suite where an angiogram confirmed severe vasospasm. As the interventionalist threaded the catheter into the right ICA, the artery clamped down and caused the $PbtO_2$ to decrease to 1.5 mm Hg. Immediate injection of intra-arterial verapamil caused vasodilatation of the right ICA and ACA distribution. The $PbtO_2$ increased to 30 mm Hg after the treatment.

Vignette 4: traumatic brain injury

PM, a 21-year-old man, sustained a severe TBI. After placement of an ICP, LICOX, and other hemodynamic lines, PM was admitted to the Neuro-Trauma ICU. After stabilization, PM's CPP decreased suddenly from 74 mm Hg to 60 mm Hg with an increase in his ICP from 21 mm Hg to 28 mm Hg. The $PbtO_2$ decreased from 26.5 mm Hg to 15.8 mm Hg. After increasing the MAP with 500 mL of albumin and drainage of CSF, the CPP increased, the ICP decreased, and the $PbtO_2$ returned to normal (Fig. 3). Optimal CPP in this patient was determined to be approximately 75 mm Hg.

In both cases, hemodynamic variables were used to optimize $PbtO_2$. Treating the underlying cause is imperative in determining the optimal CPP.

Cerebral variables, events, and interventions

Normal ICP is 0 to 15 mm Hg. An ICP of greater than 20 mm Hg is considered to be elevated and requires treatment. Increases in ICP reduce blood delivery to the brain. Studies that explored the impact of refractory increased ICP on $PbtO_2$ showed a decrease in the $PbtO_2$ when ICP was elevated significantly [52,53,63,73–75]. Strategies to reduce increased ICP include CSF drainage; head of bed elevation; neck position midline; hyperventilation; optimizing CPP; and administering medications, such as Mannitol, hypertonic saline, sedatives, analgesics, neuromuscular blockade, or pentobarbital [76]. Critical care teams should have an organized plan to reduce ICP. The influence of pentobarbital coma was reported in a case series of three patients; $PbtO_2$ was increased significantly after the induction of pentobarbital coma [73]. Two papers reported decreases in ICP and increases in $PbtO_2$ after decompressive craniectomy procedures [74,75].

Interventions to decrease an elevated ICP may help to improve the $PbtO_2$. In vignette 2 the consequence of a change in ventilator settings on ICP and $PbtO_2$ illustrated the complexity of the patient's management. Another example of the ICP–$PbtO_2$ relationship is presented in the next vignette.

Vignette 5: traumatic brain injury

AB, a 37-year-old man, sustained a severe TBI in a motorcycle accident. Cardiopulmonary resuscitation was started just as the ambulance arrived at the hospital and continued for 4 minutes. Restoration of pulses occurred. The patient was intubated and resuscitated in the ED. He went to the operating room where a large subdural hematoma was evacuated and a torn left ICA was ligated. AB was admitted to the ICU after placement of an ICP, LICOX, and other hemodynamic monitoring lines. He sustained intense periods of increased ICP that correlated with low

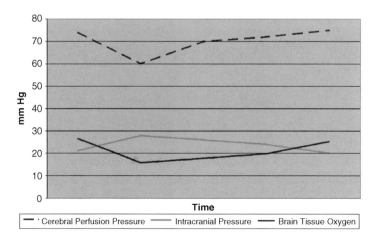

Fig. 3. CPP, ICP and $PbtO_2$ response.

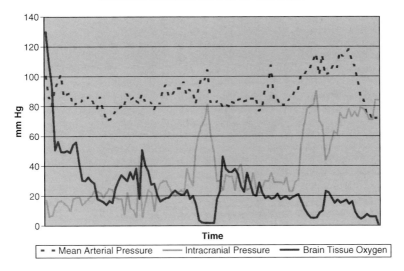

Fig. 4. Development of refractory increased ICP with decrease of PbtO$_2$.

PbtO$_2$ values. On day 3, AB's ICP increased to 85 mm Hg and exceeded his MAP. All medical and surgical interventions were used in an attempt to control the ICP. Pentobarbital coma and bilateral craniectomies were performed in an attempt to reduce the ICP. Because all interventions were exhausted, his PbtO$_2$, which had been declining with the elevated ICP, hit 0 mm Hg (Fig. 4). A bedside nuclear blood flow study was done and confirmed no CBF. The patient was pronounced brain dead. In this case,

the patient was refractory to all medical and surgical interventions that were used to reduce the increased ICP. The eventual increase of the ICP, which exceeded the MAP, led to the absence of CBF and neuronal cell death.

Vignette 6: traumatic brain injury

RH, a 39-year-old man, sustained a severe TBI in an automobile accident. He was intubated in the ED and had his intravenous lines, Foley catheter, and

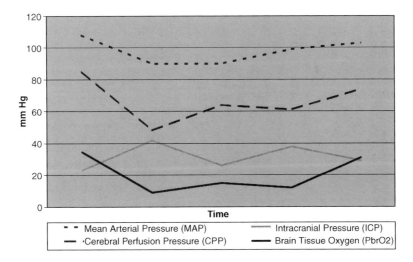

Fig. 5. Relationship of ICP, CPP, and PbtO$_2$ in a patient when neck is turned 90° in preparation for a craniectomy and then returned to the neutral position.

oral gastric tube placed. A scan of the brain showed a large subdural hematoma, intracerebral contusions, a left to right shift of the brain, and cerebral edema. RH underwent surgery for removal of a left subdural hematoma. In the operating room the surgeons placed an ICP, LICOX, and hemodynamic lines. He was admitted to the ICU for care. On the night of day 2, RH's ICP had become difficult to control, despite CSF drainage, CO_2 titrated to 33 mm Hg, CPP optimized at 80 mm Hg, Mannitol bolus given twice over 2 hours, sedation, and analgesia. His ICP hovered in the middle to high twenties. The neurosurgeon elected to take RH for a decompressive craniectomy. As the neurosurgeon was scrubbing, the operating room nurse turned the patient's neck 90° lateral to shave and prepare the scalp. Immediately, the ICP increased to 42 mm Hg, MAP/CPP decreased, and $PbtO_2$ decreased to 9 mm Hg (Fig. 5). The anesthesiologist and ICU nurses tried CSF drainage, increasing the vasopressor, and increasing the propofol to no avail. The neurosurgical clinical nurse specialist came into the room, noted the patient's position, and instructed the operating room nurse to turn the neck back to the neutral position. Upon the neck's return to the correct position, the ICP decreased to 25 mm Hg and the $PbtO_2$ increased to 27 mm Hg. The surgery was performed, and the decompressive craniectomy was effective in reducing the ICP to less than 20 mm Hg while the $PbtO_2$ maintained in the normal range.

In most clinical situations, interventions to reduce or control elevated ICP are effective. Monitoring the $PbtO_2$ adds another dimension to consider when planning interventions to control ICP.

Summary

The goal of the critical care team is to detect ischemic insults and to intervene with the most appropriate actions to restore the delivery of oxygen to the brain. The application of brain tissue oxygen monitoring technology gives practitioners another piece of information with which to make decisions when managing patients who have TBI or SAH. Properly placed brain tissue oxygen probes provide continuous data on regional oxygenation. Detecting decreases in the $PbtO_2$ and identifying the primary cause of the decline provide direction for the critical care team. Altering pulmonary, hemodynamic, and cerebral variables may enhance the delivery of oxygenated blood to the brain, and thus, ameliorate ischemic events.

References

[1] Meixenberger J, Jager A, Dings J, et al. Multimodality hemodynamic neuromonitoring—quality and consequences for therapy of severely head injured patients. Acta Neurochir (Wien) 1998;71:260–2.
[2] Jeremitsky E, Omert L, Dunham M, et al. Harbingers of poor outcome the day after severe brain injury: hypothermia, hypoxia, and hypoperfusion. J Trauma 2003;54:312–9.
[3] Vajkoczy P, Horn P, Thome C, et al. Regional cerebral blood flow monitoring in the diagnosis of delayed ischemia following aneurysmal subarachnoid hemorrhage. J Neurosurg 2003;98:1237–43.
[4] Meixensberger J, Joeger M, Voth A, et al. Brain tissue oxygen guided treatment supplementing ICP/CPP therapy after traumatic brain injury. J Neurol Neurosurg Psychiatry 2003;74:760–4.
[5] Soehle M, Jaeger M, Meixensberger J. Online assessment of brain tissue oxygen Autoregulation in traumatic brain injury and subarachnoid hemorrhage. Neurol Res 2003;254:411–7.
[6] Kett-White R, Hutchinson P, Al-Rawi P, et al. Cerebral oxygen and microdialysis monitoring during aneurysm surgery: effects of blood pressure, cerebrospinal fluid drainage, and temporary clipping on infarction. J Neurosurg 2002;96:1013–9.
[7] Andrews P. Potential end points of treatment after acute brain injury: should we be using monitors of metabolism? Curr Opin Crit Care 2003;9:83–5.
[8] Chesnut R. Management of brain and spine injuries. Crit Care Clin 2004;20:25–55.
[9] Mulvey J, Dorsch N, Mudaliar Y, et al. Multimodality monitoring in severe traumatic brain injury: the role of brain tissue oxygen monitoring. Neurocrit Care 2004;3:391–402.
[10] Dutton R, McCunn M. Traumatic brain injury. Curr Opin Crit Care 2003;9:503–9.
[11] Martin N, Patwardhan R, Alexander M, et al. Characterization of cerebral hemodynamic phases following severe head trauma: hypoperfusion, hyperemia, and vasospasm. J Neurosurg 1997;87:9–19.
[12] Bouma G, Muizelaar J. Cerebral blood flow, cerebral blood volume, and cerebrovascular reactivity after severe head injury. J Neurotrauma 1992;9(Suppl 1):S333–48.
[13] Marion D, Darby J, Yonas H. Acute regional cerebral blood flow changes caused by severe head injuries. J Neurosurg 1991;74:407–14.
[14] Bouma G, Muizelaar J. Cerebral blood flow in severe clinical head injury. New Horiz 1995;3:384–94.
[15] Lang E, Czosnyka M, Mehdorn M. Tissue oxygen reactivity and cerebral autoregulation after traumatic brain injury. Crit Care Med 2003;31:267–71.
[16] Gracias V, Guillamondegui O, Stiefel M, et al. Cerebral cortical oxygenation: a pilot study. J Trauma 2004;56:469–74.
[17] van den Brink W, van Santbrink H, Steyerberg E, et al. Brain oxygen tension in severe head injury. Neurosurgery 2000;46:868–78.

[18] Chesnut R, Marshall L, Klauber M, et al. The role of secondary brain injury in determining outcome from severe head injury. J Trauma 1993;34(2):216–22.

[19] Jones P, Andrew P, Midgley S, et al. Measuring the burden of secondary insults in head-injured patients during intensive care. J Neurosurg Anesthesiol 1994;6: 4–8.

[20] Jiang J, Gao G, Li W, et al. Early indicators of prognosis in 846 cases of severe traumatic brain injury. J Neurotrauma 2002;19:869–74.

[21] Stochetti N, Furlon A, Violta F. Hypoxemia and arterial hypotension at the accident scene in head injury. J Trauma 1996;40:764–7.

[22] Manley G, Knudson M, Morabito D, et al. Hypotension, hypoxia and head injury. Arch Surg 2001;10: 1118–23.

[23] Barton C, Hemphill J, Morabito D, et al. A novel method of evaluating the impact of secondary brain insults on functional outcomes in traumatic brain-injured patients. Acad Emerg Med 2005;12:1–6.

[24] Chesnut R, Marshall S, Pick J, et al. Early and late systemic hypotension as a frequent and fundamental source of cerebral ischemia following severe brain injury in the Traumatic Coma Data Bank. Acta Neurochir Suppl (Wien) 1993;59:121–5.

[25] Sarrafzadeh A, Peltonen E, Kaisers U, et al. Secondary insults in severe head injury—do multiply injured patients do worse? Crit Care Med 2003;29:1116–23.

[26] Coles J, Minhas P, Fryer T, et al. Effect of hyperventilation on cerebral blood flow in traumatic head injury: clinical relevance and monitoring correlates. Crit Care Med 2002;30:1950–9.

[27] Schneider G, Sarrafzadeh A, Kiening K, et al. Influence of hyperventilation on brain tissue-PO2, PCO2 and pH in patients with intracranial hypertension. Acta Neurochir Suppl 1998;71:62–5.

[28] Imberti R, Bellinzona G, Langer M. Cerebral tissue PO2 and SjvO2 changes during moderate hyperventilation in patients with severe traumatic brain injury. J Neurosurg 2002;96:97–102.

[29] van den Brink W, Santbrink H, Avezaat C, et al. Monitoring brain oxygen tension in severe head injury: The Rotterdam Experience. Acta Neurochir Suppl 1998;71:190–4.

[30] Young B, Ott L, Dempsey R, et al. Relationship between admission hyperglycemia and neurologic outcome of severely brain-injured patients. Ann Surg 1989;210(4):466–72.

[31] Lam A, Winn H, Cullen B, et al. Hyperglycemia and neurological outcome in patients with head injury. J Neurosurg 1991;75(4):545–51.

[32] Rovlias A, Kotson S. The influence of hyperglycemia on neurological outcome in patients with severe head injury. Neurosurgery 2000;46(2):335–42.

[33] Springborg J, Frederiksen H, Eskese V, et al. Trends in monitoring patients with aneurysmal subarachnoid hemorrhage. Br J Anaesth 2005;94(3):259–70.

[34] Frykholm P, Andersson J, Langstrom V, et al. Haemodynamic and metabolic disturbances in the acute stage of subarachnoid haemorrhage demonstrated by PET. Acta Neurol Scand 2004;109:25–32.

[35] Haitsma I, Maas A. Advanced monitoring in the intensive care unit: brain tissue oxygen tension. Curr Opin Crit Care 2002;8:115–20.

[36] Nemani V, Manley G. Brain tissue oxygen monitoring: physiologic principles and clinical application. Oper Tech Neurosurg 2004;7:2–9.

[37] Gesellschaft fur Medizinische Sondentechnik mbH. LICOX CMP Brain Oxygen Monitoring System Operations Manual. Plainsboro (NJ): Integra Neurosciences; 2002.

[38] Integra Neurosciences. LICOX IMC complete neuromonitoring—directions for use. Model IP2.P. Plainsboro (NJ): Integra Neurosciences; 2004.

[39] Bruzzone P, Dionigi R, Bellinzonna G, et al. Effects of cerebral perfusion pressure on brain tissue PO2 in patients with severe head injury. Acta Neurochir Suppl (Wien) 1998;71:111–3.

[40] Dings J, Meixenberger J, Amschler J, et al. Brain tissue PO2 in relation to cerebral perfusion pressure, TCD findings and TCD-CO2-reactivity after severe head injury. Acta Neurochir 1996;138:425–34.

[41] van Santbrink H, Maas A, Avezaat C. Continuous monitoring of partial pressure of brain tissue oxygen in patients with severe head injury. Neurosurgery 1996; 38:21–31.

[42] Kiening K, Unterberg A, Bardt T, et al. Monitoring of cerebral oxygenation in patients with severe head injuries: brain tissue PO2 versus jugular vein oxygen saturation. J Neurosurg 1996;85:751–7.

[43] Dings J, Meixenberger J, Jager A, et al. Clinical experience with 118 brain tissue oxygen partial pressure catheter probes. Neurosurgery 1998;43(5):1082–95.

[44] Sarrafzadeh AS, Kiening T, Bardt T, et al. Cerebral oxygenation in contusioned vs. nonlesioned brain tissue: monitoring of PtiO2 with Licox and Paratrend. Acta Neurochir Suppl 1998;71:186–9.

[45] Valadka A, Gopinath S, Contant C, et al. Relationship of brain tissue oxygen to outcome after severe head injury. Crit Care Med 1998;26:1576–81.

[46] Hoffman W, Charbel F, Edelman G. Brain tissue oxygen, carbon dioxide, and pH in neurosurgical patients at risk for ischemia. Anesth Analg 1996;82: 294–301.

[47] Zauner A, Doppenberg E, Young H, et al. Brain oxygen monitoring predicts outcome after severe head injury. Journal of Neurotrauma 1996;13:619.

[48] Doppenberg E, Zauner A, Bullock R, et al. Correlations between brain tissue oxygen tension, carbon dioxide tension, pH and cerebral blood flow—a better way of monitoring the severely injured brain? Surg Neurol 1998;49(6):650–4.

[49] Maas A, Fleckenstein W, de Jong D, et al. Monitoring cerebral oxygenation: experimental studies and preliminary clinical results of continuous monitoring of cerebrospinal fluid and brain tissue oxygen tension. Acta Neurochir Suppl (Wein) 1993;59:50–7.

[50] Meixensberger J, Dings J, Kuhnig H, et al. Studies

of tissue PO2 in normal and pathological human brain cortex. Acta Neurochir Suppl (Wien) 1993;59:58–63.

[51] Hlatky R, Valadka A, Robertson C. Intracranial hypertension and cerebral ischemia after severe traumatic brain injury. Neurosurg Focus 2003;14:1–4.

[52] Bardt T, Unterberg A, Hartl R, et al. Monitoring of brain tissue PO2 in traumatic brain injury: effect of cerebral hypoxia on outcome. Acta Neurochir Suppl 1998;71:153–6.

[53] Palmer S, Bader MK. Brain tissue oxygenation in brain death. Neurocrit Care 2005;2:17–22.

[54] McCance K, Huether S. Pathophysiology: the biologic basis for disease in adults and children. St. Louis (MO): Mosby Inc.; 2002.

[55] Yundt K, Kiringer M. The use of hyperventilation and its impact on cerebral ischemia in the treatment of traumatic brain injury. Crit Care Clin 1997;13:163–83.

[56] March K, Wellwood J. Intracranial pressure concepts and cerebral blood flow. In: Bader MK, Littlejohns L, editors. AANN core curriculum for neuroscience nursing. 4th edition. St. Louis (MO): Elsevier; 2004.

[57] Johnston A, Steiner L, Gupta A, et al. Cerebral oxygen vasoreactivity and cerebral tissue oxygen reactivity. Br J Anesth 2003;90:774–86.

[58] Gopinath S, Valadka A, Uzura M, et al. Comparison of jugular venous oxygen saturation and brain tissue PO2 as monitors of cerebral ischemia after head injury. Neurosurgical Intensive Care 1999;27:2337–45.

[59] Menzel M, Doppenberg E, Zauner A, et al. Increased inspired oxygen concentration as a factor in improved brain tissue oxygenation and tissue lactate levels after severe human head injury. J Neurosurg 1999;91:1–10.

[60] Tolias C, Reinert M, Seiler R, et al. Normobaric hyperoxia-induced improvement in cerebral metabolism and reduction in intracranial pressure in patients with severe head injury: a prospective historical cohort-matched study. J Neurosurg 2004;101:435–44.

[61] Reinert M, Barth A, Rothen H, et al. Effects of cerebral perfusion pressure and increased fraction of inspired oxygen on brain tissue oxygen, lactate, and glucose in patients with severe head injury. Acta Neurochir (Wien) 2003;145:341–50.

[62] Magnoni S, Ghisoni L, Locatelli M, et al. Lack of improvement in cerebral metabolism after hyperoxia in severe head injury: a microdialysis study. J Neurosurg 2003;98:952–8.

[63] Kiening K, Hartl R, Unterberg A, et al. Brain tissue pO2 monitoring in comatose patients: implications for therapy. Journal of Neurologic Research 1997;19:1–8.

[64] Gupta A, Hutchinson P, Al-Rawi P, et al. Measuring brain tissue oxygenation compared with jugular venous oxygen saturation for monitoring cerebral oxygenation after traumatic brain injury. Anesth Analg 1999;88:549–53.

[65] Reinprecht A, Greher M, Wolfsberger S, et al. Prone positioning in subarachnoid hemorrhage patients with acute respiratory distress syndrome: effects on cerebral tissue oxygenation and intracranial pressure. Crit Care Med 2003;31:1831–8.

[66] Smith M, Stiefel M, Magge S, et al. Packed red blood cell transfusion increases local cerebral oxygenation. Crit Care Med 2005;33:1104–8.

[67] Vespa P. What is the optimal threshold for cerebral perfusion pressure following traumatic brain injury? Neurosurg Focus 2003;15:1–5.

[68] Stochetti N, Chieregato A, De Marchi M, et al. High cerebral perfusion pressure improves low values of local brain tissue O2 tension in focal lesions. Acta Neurochir Suppl 1998;71:162–5.

[69] Johnston A, Steiner L, Coles J, et al. Effect of cerebral perfusion pressure autoregulation on regional oxygenation and metabolism after head injury. Crit Care Med 2005;33:189–95.

[70] Charbel F, Du X, Hoffman W, et al. Brain tissue PO2, PCO2, and pH during cerebral vasospasm. Surg Neurol 2000;54:432–8.

[71] Hoelper B, Hofmann E, Sporleder R, et al. Transluminal balloon angioplasty improves brain tissue oxygenation and metabolism in severe vasospasm after aneurysmal subarachnoid hemorrhage: Case report. Neurosurgery 2003;52:970–6.

[72] Stiefel M, Heuer G, Abrahams J, et al. The effect of nimodipine on cerebral oxygenation in patients with poor grade subarachnoid hemorrhage. J Neurosurg 2004;101:594–9.

[73] McKinley B, Parmley C. Effects of injury and therapy on brain parenchyma pO2, PCO2, pH, and ICP following severe closed head injury. Acta Neurochir Suppl 1998;71:177–82.

[74] Jaeger M, Soehle M, Meixensberger J. Effects of decompressive craniectomy on brain tissue oxygen in patients with intracranial hypertension. J Neurol Neurosurg Psychiatry 2003;74:513–5.

[75] Stiefel M, Heuer G, Smith M, et al. Cerebral oxygenation following decompressive craniectomy for the treatment of refractory intracranial pressure. J Neurosurg 2004;101:241–7.

[76] Dunn L. Raised intracranial pressure. J Neurol Neurosurg Psychiatry 2002;73:23–7.

CRITICAL CARE
NURSING CLINICS
OF NORTH AMERICA

Crit Care Nurs Clin N Am 18 (2006) 257–265

Glycemic Control After Coronary Bypass Graft: Using Intravenous Insulin Regulated by a Computerized System

Elaine Button, RN, CDE*, Patty Keaton, RN, BSN, CCRN

Moses Cone Health System, 1200 North Elm Street, Greensboro, NC 27401, USA

Hyperglycemia is a risk factor for poor outcomes in patients who undergo coronary artery bypass grafting (CABG) [1–9]. Poor outcomes, such as sepsis, nosocomial infections, deep sternal wound infections, increased mortality, renal failure, and polyneuropathy, led a multidisciplinary team to formulate a protocol to improve the glycemic control of inpatients who had diabetes or hyperglycemia. This protocol initiated an intravenous (IV) insulin infusion that is regulated by a computerized system that is known as a Glucommander, and guides the surgeon and nurses to an easy transition to subcutaneous insulin. As a result of implementing the computerized system glycemic control improved during surgery and postoperatively. Additionally, physician and nurse satisfaction increased.

The prevalence of diabetes in the United States has increased 33% over the last 8 years according to the Centers for Disease Control and Prevention [10]. As many as 1.5 million patients are hospitalized with significant hyperglycemia and no history of diabetes [11]. Data show that treating hyperglycemia—regardless of the cause—early and aggressively can reduce mortality, morbidity, length of hospital stay, and medical costs [1–9,11]. Thirty-six percent of all patients who undergo CABG have a diagnosis of diabetes. Guidelines by the American College of Endocrinologists recommend a target blood glucose of 110 mg/dL in the ICU population [12]. Sternal wound infection is a common complication in patients who have diabetes and who undergo CABG [1–4]. As

more data has focused on the negative effects of hyperglycemia, emphasis has been placed on the need for aggressive management of blood glucose levels in patients who undergo open heart surgery.

The Diabetes Treatment Program (DTP) staff at Moses Cone Memorial Hospital observed that approximately 90% of patients who had diabetes who had CABG surgery had elevated blood glucose levels (200–300 mg/dL) when they arrived in the surgical ICU (SICU) postoperatively. At that time the surgeon would order an IV insulin drip without any protocol. This required the critical care nurse to make frequent phone calls to the physician for adjustment or verification of the drip rate. Transitioning from IV to subcutaneous insulin was hit and miss and resulted in patients being transferred out of the SICU with less than optimal control (Fig. 1). The cardiovascular thoracic (CVT) surgeons wanted better glycemic control and so did the nurses. ICU nurses played a key role in making the decision to improve glycemic control and were instrumental in the development of the protocol and use of the computerized tool [13]. A blood glucose level of greater than 200 mg/dL postoperatively for patients who had undergone CABG was identified as a problem.

A multidisciplinary team was formed to address glycemic control in the CABG population. Key players on the team included cardiovascular surgeons, a pharmacist, SICU staff nurses, DTP inpatient director, a clinician, and the medical director. The goal of the team was to reduce glucose levels intraoperatively and postoperatively, and to maintain blood glucose levels at less than 150 mg/dL during the ICU stay. Primary quality issues that were identified by the team included lack of standardization of periopera-

---

* Corresponding author.

E-mail address: elaine.button@mosescone.com
(E. Button).

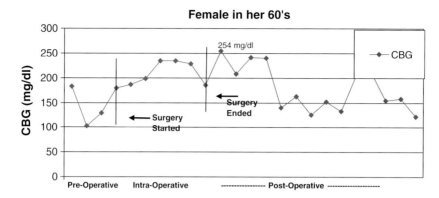

Fig. 1. Capillary blood glucose level in a woman in her sixties who underwent CABG. She had no IV insulin during surgery or postoperatively.

tive care for diabetic or hyperglycemic patients who underwent open heart surgery; lack of consistent testing and documentation of hourly capillary blood glucose (CBG) levels immediately before the surgery, during surgery, and after surgery; treatment of hyperglycemia during the intraoperative period; and lack of consistent transition from IV to subcutaneous insulin.

The use of IV insulin is imperative in the ICU for safe and efficient glycemic control. [1,3–9] Titration and regulation of the insulin drip often is difficult to maintain and achieve. The new protocol used a tool called the Glucommander to assist in initiation and maintenance of insulin drip rates based on a computerized algorithm.

Glucommander

The Glucommander is a computerized algorithm system that is used to resolve hyperglycemia and to maintain normoglycemia in the acute hospital setting. It is used in combination with, but independently of, an IV insulin drip and a bedside glucose monitor. The Glucommander program is installed on a small laptop computer. The physician orders the use of the Glucommander and the key components, which are entered into the program. The parameters that are ordered by the physician include low and high blood glucose targets and an initial multiplier. After the initial multiplier is entered, the computer calculates subsequent multipliers based on the patient's response to the insulin infusion as indicated by CBGs entered in the Glucommander screen. Glucose measurements are requested (by an alarm) at intervals that range from 20 minutes to a maximum interval that

is prescribed by the physician. The software determines the interval between measurements based on the stability of the blood glucose levels of the patient. The insulin infusion rate adjustment is based on the glucose value entered into the software and

Table 1
Example of the amount of IV insulin required as dictated by the Glucommander

Location	Time	Glucose (mg/dL)	Insulin drip (units/h)	Subcutaneous insulin
OR	2100	227	11.2	
	2200	187	12.2	
	2300	165	11.6	
	2400	157	12	
	0100	134	10	
	0200	121	8.7	
	0300	151	6.3	
	0400	126	9.0	
SICU	0500	108	8.0	
	0600	115	7.6	
	0700	100	Drip discontinued	
	0800	89	No insulin required	
	1000	100	No insulin required	
	1200	120		NovoLog 2 units
	1600	159		NovoLog 2 units
	2000	188		NovoLog 4 units
	2200			Lantus 50 units

Women in her forties who had type 1 diabetes who underwent emergency CABG with four grafts.
Abbreviation: OR, operating room.

the slope of the blood glucose curve. The nurse adjusts the patient's IV insulin infusion based on the rate indicated on the Glucommander screen (Table 1). Some of the safety features of the Glucommander include:

All blood glucose levels are entered twice.

The highest blood glucose that can be entered is 999, which will set the maximum amount of insulin.

The multiplier is adjusted up or down based on the slope of the blood glucose curve between readings and the initial parameters set by the physician. If the blood glucose is within target range the multiplier remains unchanged.

The Glucommander alarms hourly to remind the practitioner to check and enter the current

CBG level. If the blood glucose is low or decreasing faster than expected, the program can alarm every 20 minutes for insulin drip adjustment. If the blood glucose is within target range for 5 consecutive readings the Glucommander alarms every 2 hours.

Protocol development

The team's strategies for protocol development included implementing a system to identify patients who had diabetes and hyperglycemia before they underwent CABG. IV insulin infusion that was regulated by the Glucommander was initiated at the start of surgery (Fig. 2). In the first order set, patients were

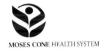

MOSES CONE HEALTH SYSTEM

Glucommander Standards or Care Orders for patients with diabetes who have CABG.

Use the following settings for all CVTS CABG patients with diabetes:

1. Low Value Target Range   100
2. High Value Target Range   150
3. Maximum Minutes for checking blood glucose   60
4. Initial Multiplier   .03
5. Number of units of insulin per CC.   1

Physician's signatures:

_____ Date_____
_____ Date_____
_____ Date_____
_____ Date_____
_____ Date_____

Fig. 2. Preoperative protocol. (Courtesy of Moses Cone Health System, Greensboro, NC; with permission.)

MOSES CONE HEALTH SYSTEM **PHYSICIAN'S ORDERS**

	DATE	TIME		
START HERE →			DRUG SENSITIVITY	* A GENERICALLY OR THERAPEUTICALLY EQUIVALENT DRUG AS APPROVED BY THE PHARMACY COMMITTEE MAY BE DISPENSED UNLESS OTHERWISE SPECIFICALLY STATED.
				1.
				2.
				3.
				4.

Cardiac Surgery Diabetes Patients Only
IV to Subcutaneous INSULIN Orders
(Renal patients may require less insulin)

1. Suspend IV insulin drip when one or more or the following occurs:
   A. Patient is eating, **or**
   B. Insulin drip has been titrated down to 1 unit/hour, **or**
   C. Blood sugar is <90mg/dl.
2. Give Glargine / Lantus® per orders below [#5A or 5B].
3. Continue to check blood sugar q1h <u>and</u> infuse IV insulin per Glucommander x 3 hours, then discontinue Glucommander and IV insulin drip.
4. Start sliding scale as indicated below [#6] after IV drip discontinued.

5. <u>A.   For Type 1 patients</u>:
   Give Glargine / Lantus® INSULIN (0.1-0.2 units/kg) _____units subcutaneous X 1dose.
   <u>B.   For Type 2 patients</u>:
   Give Glargine / Lantus® INSULIN (0.3-0.4 units/kg) _____units subcutaneous X 1dose.

   ### *[DO NOT MIX Glargine / Lantus® with any other insulin]*.

6. Start CVTS Regular insulin sliding scale q_____hrs as indicated after Glucommander discontinued.

000-149 mg/dl = 00	units subcutaneous or _____units.
150-200 mg/dl = 04	units subcutaneous or _____units.
201-250 mg/dl = 08	units subcutaneous or _____units.
251-300 mg/dl = 12	units subcutaneous or _____units.
301-350 mg/dl = 16	units subcutaneous or _____units.
351-450 mg/dl = 20	units subcutaneous or _____units.
>451 mg/dl = 24	units subcutaneous, plus obtain a STAT GLUCOSE and Notify MD.

NURSING SECRETARY _____   R.N. _____   PHYSICIAN _____ DATE _____

MR91191(8/01)   White – CHART   Yellow – PHARMACY   Pink – NURSING

Fig. 3. Physician's orders form for diabetic patients who are undergoing cardiac surgery, Version 1. (Courtesy of Moses Cone Health System, Greensboro, NC; with permission.)

MOSES CONE HEALTH SYSTEM **PHYSICIAN'S ORDERS**

* A GENERICALLY OR THERAPEUTICALLY EQUIVALENT DRUG AS APPROVED BY THE
PHARMACY COMMITTEE MAY BE DISPENSED UNLESS OTHERWISE SPECIFICALLY STATED.

START HERE →	DATE	TIME	DRUG SENSITIVITY	1.
				2.
				3.
				4.

Cardiac Surgery Diabetes Patients Only
IV to Subcutaneous INSULIN Orders
(Renal patients may require less insulin)

1. On admission to SICU, continue IV insulin drip per Glucommander to maintain CBG between 90 and 120 mg/dl.
2. Continue IV insulin drip per Glucommander until CBG is below 120 mg/dl x 3 consecutive hourly readings.
3. When CBG is below 120 mg/dl x 3 hours, stop IV insulin drip/Glucommander and start **CVTS insulin sliding scale 1 hour after IV is discontinued.**
4. Check CBG q 2 hours x 3, then q 4 hours. Patient may advance to ac & hs when eating. Give sliding scale insulin as needed after each CBG check.
5. At 2200 (10pm), give Glargine / Lantus® per orders below [A or B].

Glargine / Lantus® Insulin orders
A. Patients with no pharmacologic therapy or patients on insulin alone prior to admission: (0.2 units - 0.4 units/kg) _____ units subcutaneous.
B. Patients on oral therapy or oral/insulin therapy prior to admission:
                (0.4 units/kg) _____ units subcutaneous.

DO NOT MIX Glargine / Lantus® in the same syringe with any other insulin.

Humalog / Novolog Insulin Sliding Scale
000-119 mg/dl = 00 units subcutaneous or	_____ units.
120-160 mg/dl = 02 units subcutaneous or	_____ units.
161-200 mg/dl = 04 units subcutaneous or	_____ units.
201-250 mg/dl = 08 units subcutaneous or	_____ units.
251-300 mg/dl = 12 units subcutaneous or	_____ units.
301-350 mg/dl = 16 units subcutaneous or	_____ units.
351-450 mg/dl = 20 units subcutaneous or	_____ units.
>451 mg/dl = 24 units subcutaneous, plus obtain a STAT GLUCOSE and and Notify MD.	

NURSING SECRETARY   R.N.   PHYSICIAN   DATE

White – CHART   Yellow – PHARMACY

MR 91191 rev 1-03

Fig. 4. CVT surgeon's orders form for Glucommander, Version 2. (Courtesy of Moses Cone Health System, Greensboro, NC; with permission.)

MOSES CONE HEALTH SYSTEM

PHYSICIAN'S ORDERS

* A GENERICALLY OR THERAPEUTICALLY EQUIVALENT DRUG AS APPROVED BY THE
PHARMACY COMMITTEE MAY BE DISPENSED UNLESS OTHERWISE SPECIFICALLY STATED.

START HERE →	DATE	TIME	DRUG SENSITIVITY	1.
				2.
				3.
				4.

CVTS Glucommander Orders
IV to Subcutaneous INSULIN Orders
(Renal patients may require less insulin)

1. On admission to unit, continue IV insulin drip (100 units regular insulin/100 ml normal saline) per Glucommander to maintain CBG between 90 and 120 mg/dl.
[Change Glucommander low and high range, if needed to 90 to 120].

2. Continue IV insulin drip per Glucommander until CBG is below 120 mg/dl x 3 consecutive hourly readings.

3. When CBG is below 120 mg/dl x 3 hours, stop IV insulin drip/Glucommander and start **CVTS insulin sliding scale* 1 hour after IV is discontinued.**

4. Check CBG q 2 hours x 3, then q 4 hours. Give sliding scale insulin as indicated after each CBG check. If patient on pre-hospitalization Insulin and CBG greater than 200 with first q 2 hr check, then restart Glucommander per protocol with Insulin drip. DO NOT RESTART AFTER 1:00 AM.

5. When eating, advance to ac & hs CBG's and give sliding scale insulin* as indicated.

---

* CVTS Novolog Insulin Sliding Scale (Subcutaneous)

000-119 mg/dl =   0 units subcutaneous or _____ units.
120-160 mg/dl =   2 units subcutaneous or _____ units.
161-200 mg/dl =   4 units subcutaneous or _____ units.
201-250 mg/dl =   8 units subcutaneous or _____ units.
251-300 mg/dl = 12 units subcutaneous or _____ units.
301-350 mg/dl = 16 units subcutaneous or _____ units.
351-450 mg/dl = 20 units subcutaneous or _____ units.
>451 mg/dl   = 24 units subcutaneous, plus obtain a STAT LAB GLUCOSE and Notify MD.

---

6. At 2200 (10 PM), give initial Glargine (Lantus®) per orders below [A or B].**

** Initial Glargine (Lantus®) Insulin orders

A. <u>Patients with no hypoglycemic therapy or patients on insulin alone prior to admission:</u>
(0.2 units - 0.4 units/kg) _____ units subcutaneous.

B. <u>Patients on oral hypoglycemic therapy or oral hypoglycemic/insulin therapy prior to admission:</u>
(0.4 units - 0.5 units/kg) _____ units subcutaneous.
DO NOT MIX Glargine (Lantus®) with any other insulin.

NURSING SECRETARY _____   R.N. _____   PHYSICIAN _____   DATE _____

MR91191 (2/04)   White – CHART   Yellow – PHARMACY

Fig. 5. CVT surgeon's (CVTS) postoperative orders form for transition from IV to subcutaneous insulin, Version 3. (Courtesy of Moses Cone Health System, Greensboro, NC; with permission.)

given basal insulin when the criteria for discontinuing the IV insulin drip (patient is eating or insulin drip was titrated to 1 unit/h or blood glucose was less than 90 mg/dL) were met (Fig. 3). Basal insulin was given 3 hours after the criteria were met. Blood glucose levels were checked every hour for 3 hours and then the sliding scale insulin was given as needed. In the second version of the order set, the target range for blood glucose in the SICU was changed to 90 to 120 mg/dL. Patients continued on the insulin drip postoperatively in the SICU until three consecutive hourly CBG levels were within target range. Transition to subcutaneous basal insulin occurred based on weight (Fig. 4). The third version of the orders increased the glargine dosage to a maximum of 0.5 units/kg (Fig. 5).

The Glucommander settings were discussed and decided upon by the multidisciplinary team. Initially, the target range of 100 to 150 mg/dL initially was programmed into the Glucommander. This range resulted in a significant improvement and reduced the fear of hypoglycemia for the anesthetized patient. The CVT surgeons chose 0.3 as the initial multiplier based on the resistance of insulin common in the CABG population and type 2 diabetes. The CVT surgeons added A1C to the order set to determine the duration of the hyperglycemia and previous glycemic control. Based on the A1C results and the patient's educational needs, the CVT surgeons also encouraged and ordered outpatient diabetes education 4 to 6 weeks after discharge.

After the initial protocol was developed and put into print, training included the disciplines that are involved with the use of the IV insulin drip/Glucommander. This training was done with the anesthesiologists, nurse anesthetists, IV perfusion team, SICU nurses, presurgical RN team, pharmacists, and CVT surgeons. A pilot was conducted for 1 month to determine the effectiveness of the protocol. Objectives of the protocol were:

- Hourly blood glucose checks at the beginning of surgery and throughout the intraoperative period
- IV insulin drip bags were mixed by the pharmacy for all patients who had diabetes, and were sent to the preoperative holding area with the other IV solutions and medications
- Glucose levels reduced to less than 150 mg/dL during the intraoperative and postoperative period
- Subcutaneous insulin was given before the IV insulin drip was discontinued, and a basal insulin was initiated as part of the transition from IV to subcutaneous insulin

Barriers

System barriers were identified and addressed to assure success of the glycemic control interventions. These barriers included the timely delivery of IV insulin drip to the operating room by the pharmacy, the potential for increased costs associated with the increased number of finger sticks for CBG or by a portable chemistry analyzer (iSTAT) that were performed, and the staff's resistance to checking hourly CBG levels. Each barrier was addressed openly with the multidisciplinary team and was addressed separately with each discipline to the satisfaction of the majority. Addressing the barriers took time and delayed implementation, but it was important to have support from the key users. One of the most effective strategies was the one-to-one demonstration of the Glucommander with the Anesthesia Department. The DTP clinicians spent several days in the Anesthesia lounge demonstrating the Glucommander to the certified nurse anesthetists. The informal setting was conducive to increased dialog, and provided a forum for uncovering obstacles and addressing misperceptions regarding the use of the Glucommander. An additional benefit of the intensive training was the identification of individuals who were interested in this new tool and who were willing to use it. Initially, the Anesthesia Department was skeptical about whether the IV insulin would be available at the beginning of surgery, and whether they would be able to fit another hourly test into their heavy schedule. They also questioned whether this tool would be effective and safe. The outcomes proved beneficial. Four years later the Glucommander is standard procedure with all patients who undergo CABG and who experience hyperglycemia.

Transitioning patients from intravenous to subcutaneous insulin

Transitioning the patient from IV to subcutaneous insulin was, and continues to be, the greatest challenge. When the patient is not eating and is on IV insulin, managing glycemic control is easy. When food, total nutrition alimentation, or increased activity is introduced, the challenge is to find the perfect subcutaneous dosage and timing of insulin to anticipate the physiologic needs of each person. In addition, patients may be nauseated one day and feel better the next with varying amounts of activity and food consumption. Further, if the patient has not been on insulin previously the dilemma is which insulin to use and the correct dosage. Should the cost of the insulin be a consideration?

Table 2
Key revisions to the postoperative orders

Key orders	Order set #1	Order set #2	Order set #3
IV insulin discontinued	When one of the following occurred: -Patient eating -Insulin drip @ 1 unit/h -CBG <90 mg/dL	When three consecutive CBGs <120 mg/dL	When three consecutive CBGs <120 mg/dL
Sliding-scale insulin	Initiated when CBG >150 mg/dL Regular insulin used	Initiated when CBG >120 mg/dL	Initiated when CBG >120 mg/dL
Glargine initiated	When one of the three criteria in section 1 met	At 2200 (10:00 PM)	At 2200 (10:00 PM)
CBG levels ordered	Dosage based on 0.1–0.4 units/kg Every 1 hour × 3, then per MD	Dosage based on 0.2–0.4 units/kg Every 2 hours × 3, then every 4 hours, then ac & hs when eating	Dosage based on 0.2–0.5 units/kg Every 2 hours × 3, then every 4 hours, then ac & hs when eating

For this project a postoperative order set was developed using a basal, peakless insulin, glargine (Lantus), which had just been approved by the U.S. Food and Drug Administration and was available in the authors' market. It had been marketed primarily as an insulin for outpatient use; however, the multidisciplinary team believed that it might work well for patients who were in the hospital (who were NPO one hour and eating the next). It provided a steady state of insulin, similar to a timed-released capsule. In hospitals, basal insulin needs often are overlooked when patients go for procedures or surgery. Glargine can provide for basal needs without causing hypoglycemia. The transition orders used the patient's weight to dose insulin glargine. Each patient was given a dosage of insulin glargine at 2200 (10:00 PM).

IV insulin was stopped when three consecutive blood sugar levels were less than 120 mg/dL. An aggressive sliding scale that used insulin aspart (NovoLog) was started when the IV insulin was discontinued. NovoLog is a rapid-acting insulin that begins working within 5 to 10 minutes after injection, peaks at 0.5 to 1.5 hours, and has an effective duration of 3 to 4 hours. When rapid-acting insulin was initiated, CBG levels were tested every 2 hours for three times and every 4 hours while in the ICU.

Key components of the transition orders included the following:

IV insulin drip was discontinued when glucose level was less than 120 mg/dL for 3 hours
All patients received basal subcutaneous insulin at bedtime (10 PM)
CBG levels were obtained within 1 hour of IV insulin discontinuation and were continued every 2 hours for 6 hours and every 4 hours thereafter
Aggressive sliding-scale coverage every 4 hours until the patient was eating
Sliding scale (correction) insulin before meals and at bedtime after the patient was eating

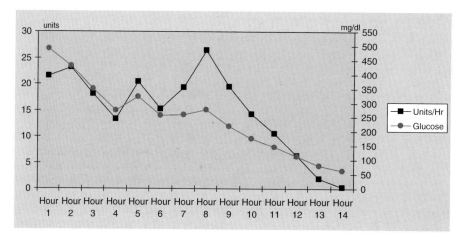

Fig. 6. Glucommander controls blood glucose with continuous automatic adjustment of insulin rate.

Less subcutaneous sliding-scale insulin was required as a result of initiating a basal insulin before the IV insulin drip was discontinued. The glycemic outcomes that were achieved with the protocol improved with each revision (Table 2).

Outcomes

Primary outcomes were impressive. Blood glucose levels were monitored and documented consistently in the operating room, and were reduced to an average of 120 mg/dL postoperatively (Fig. 6). Glycemic control was improved after the IV insulin drip was discontinued by giving a basal subcutaneous insulin before discontinuing the IV. Ancillary outcomes that resulted from the implementation of glycemic control included identification of newly diagnosed diabetics, increased outpatient diabetes education referrals, and A1C orders on all patients who had a glucose level 200 mg/dL.

Summary

This protocol was initiated for all patients who had diabetes or hyperglycemia and underwent CABG surgery. Patients were treated with an IV insulin infusion that was regulated by a computerized algorithm system, known as the Glucommander, that lasted from the onset of surgery through the postoperative period. Each patient was transitioned to subcutaneous insulin using a bedtime dose of insulin glargine and a sliding scale using insulin aspart. The result was a significant improvement in glycemic control in the SICU. Most patients had an average postoperative blood glucose level of 120 mg/dL. The benefits to the participating institution were increased awareness of the importance of improving blood glucose control, improved timeliness of transport of IV insulin to the surgical department, decreased calls to physicians, increased outpatient education referrals, decreased need for sliding-scale insulin injections, increased nursing satisfaction because of fewer calls to physicians for insulin adjustment, and increased physician satisfaction because of improved blood glucose control and fewer interruptive phone calls.

Acknowledgments

Special thanks and appreciation are due to the Diabetes Treatment Program (DTP) staff who assisted

in this project. They are: Patti Routh, RN, MSN, CDE; Ann Clark, RN, MSN, CDE; Lynn Parker, RN, CDE; Judy Hanks, RN, BSN, CDE. Jenny Simpson, RN, MSN, and Joanne Westerfield, RN, MSN, Healthways, reviewed and gave valuable input to this article. The surgical ICU staff, anesthesia staff, cardiovascular surgeons, and pharmacists were vital to the implementation and ongoing success of the project.

References

[1] Furnary AP, Zerr KJ, Grunkemeier GL, et al. Continuous intravenous insulin infusion reduces the incidence of deep sternal wound infection in diabetic patients after cardiac surgical procedures. Ann Thor Surg 1999;67(2):352–60.

[2] Umpierrez GE, Isaacs SD, Bazargan N, et al. Hyperglycemia: an independent marker of in-hospital mortality in patients with undiagnosed diabetes. J Clin Endocrinol Metab 2002;87:978–82.

[3] Furnary AP, Gao G, Grunkemeier GL, et al. Continuous insulin infusion reduces mortality in patients with diabetes undergoing coronary artery bypass grafting. J Thorac Cardiovasc Surg 2003;125:1007–21.

[4] Zerr KJ, Furnary AP, Grunkemeier GL, et al. Glucose control lowers the risk of wound infections in diabetics after open heart operations. Ann Thorac Surg 1997;63:356–61.

[5] Levetan CS. Controlling hyperglycemia in the hospital: a matter of life and death. Clin Diabetes 2002;18:17–24.

[6] Krinsley JS. Effect of an intensive glucose management protocol on the mortality of critically ill adult patients. Mayo Clin Proc 2004;79(8):992–1000.

[7] Van den Berghe G, Wouters P, Weekers F, et al. Intensive insulin therapy in critically ill patients. N Engl J Med 2001;345:1359–67.

[8] Clement S, Braithwaite SS, Magee MF, et al. Management of diabetes and hyperglycemia in hospitals. Diabetes Care 2004;27:553–79.

[9] Grey NJ, Perdrizet GA. Reduction of nosocomial infections in the surgical intensive care unit by strict glycemic control. Endocr Pract 2004;10(Suppl 2):46–52.

[10] Center for Disease Control and Prevention. National diabetes fact sheet: general information and national estimates on diabetes in the United States, revised edition. Available at: www.cdc.gov/diabetes. Accessed September 7, 2005.

[11] Unger J, Marcus AO. Glucose control in the hospitalized patient. Emerg Med 2004;36(9):12–8.

[12] American College of Endocrinology (ACE) Position Statement on Inpatient Diabetes and Metabolic Control. Endocr Pract 2004;10(Suppl 2):5–9.

[13] Roberts SR, Hamedani B. Benefits and methods of achieving strict glycemic control in the ICU. Crit Care Nurs Clin North Am 2004;16:537–45.

ELSEVIER
SAUNDERS

Crit Care Nurs Clin N Am 18 (2006) 267–271

CRITICAL CARE
NURSING CLINICS
OF NORTH AMERICA

Index

Note: Page numbers of article titles are in **boldface** type.

A

Acidosis, and secondary brain injury, 244–245

Acute coronary syndrome (ACS), continuous
ST-segment monitoring in, 170

Amiodarone, QT interval prolongation with,
161–162

Angina, variant. See *Variant angina.*

Arterial pulse technologies, applications of, clinical
importance of, 182–185
arterial waveform components in, dicrotic
notch, 181
forward flow, 181
reflective wave, 181–182
heart-lung mechanics and, impact of respiration
on, 184–185
with mechanical ventilation, 185
in cardiac output monitoring, currently available,
179–180
physiologic requirements for, 180
theory behind, 179
in evaluation of response to fluid
administration, 185
in fluid responsiveness assessment, arterial
pressure-based parameters in, 183–184
physiology supporting, 183–184
physiologic basis of, factors affecting the arterial
pulse, 181
interrelationships of pressure, resistance, and
flow, 181
respiration and, relationships between airway and
arterial pressures in, 184
theory behind, 182–183

Arterial waveform, components of, 181–182
technical factors affecting, 185–186

B

Bioimpedance cardiography, advantage of, 197–198
after cardiac transplantation, 198
current systems for, 201

devices for, thoracic, 196
variation in, 195
whole-body, 196
hemodynamic data in, 196–199
impedance technique in, 196
in prediction of heart failure events, 198–199
popularity of, reasons for, 195
pulmonary artery catheter and, 198
pulmonary artery wedge pressure and, 197
right atrial pressure in, 197
therapeutic value of, during dialysis, 200
in chronic fatigue syndrome, 200–201
in heart failure, 200
in pacing failure, 200
in peripartum women with preeclampsia, 200
in resistant hypertension, 199–200
unavailability of right arterial and pulmonary
artery wedge pressure values, 196–197
validation studies of, 201
versus pulmonary artery catheter, 196

Bispectral (BIS) index monitoring, case series with
neuromuscular blockade, decisiveness of,
237, 239
methods in, 231
patients in, 230–231
with bronchogenic lung cancer, respiratory
distress, 233, 236–237
with COPD exacerbation, 231–232
with end-stage liver disease, bleeding
esophageal varices, 233
with epiglottis, 232, 235
with ethanol/alcohol dependency
withdrawal, 233, 236
with exacerbation of COPD, progressive
respiratory failure, 232
with HIV infection, severe respiratory
failure, 233, 236
with interstitial pneumonia, AIDS, 233, 235
with PCP pneumonia, respiratory failure,
233, 235
with pneumonia, respiratory failure, 232, 235

doi:10.1016/S0899-5885(06)00041-4

response to, 147
safety standard for, 145
true *versus* false, 149–150

Clinical alarm systems, assessments of, 148–151
    activation and practice, 151
    risk associated with, 151
    Wake Medical Center tool for, 148
clinical policies and, 154–155
components of, 152–153
default settings in, 154
educational program for, 155
equipment selection for, 152
evaluation of, 153–154
metrics of success with, 155
problems with, 151–152
risk assessment of, 149–150
safety program for, 152
staff competency and, validation of, 153–154
technology and, 152–154
testing plan for, development of, 151

Congestive heart failure, continuous venous oxygen
    saturation monitoring in, 207

Continuous venous oxygen saturation (ScvO₂)
    monitoring, clinical applications of, 205–208
    early goal-directed therapy, 206
    in cardiac arrest, 207
        resuscitation period following, 207
    in cardiac surgery, 208
    in congestive heart failure, acutely
        decompensated, 207
    in sepsis and septic shock, 206–207
    in trauma and hemorrhagic shock, 208
interpretation of, 205
measurement of, 204–205
physiological relationship with mixed venous
    oxygen saturation in, 204–205

Coronary artery bypass graft (CABG), glycemic
    control following, IV insulin for, **257–265**
    in patients with diabetes, Glucommander control
        of IV insulin for, 258–262
    glycemic control following, outcomes of, 265
    protocol development for Glucommander use,
        259, 263
    transitioning from IV to subcutaneous insulin,
        263–264

D

Dead space, physiologic, 219

Dysrhythmias, ST-segment monitoring and, 171–172

E

ECG monitoring, abnormalities on, 165, 167
electrophysiologic concepts in, 166–167
    for prolonged QT interval and proarrhythmia, and
        for impending torsades de pointes, 162
    calculation of corrected QT interval, 162
    correction of QT interval for heart rate, 162
    QT-prolonging drugs and, 161–162
    recommendations for, 161
in hospital settings, practice standards for,
    157–168
interpretation of data from, staff qualifications for,
    165–167
12-lead ECG, derived *versus* standard, diagnostic
    accuracy of, 163–164
    documentation of wide QRS tachycardias and
        myocardial ischemia, 164
    limb lead placement for, 163
lead systems for, 163–165
of arrhythmia, in hospital settings, **157–168**
    nursing responsibilities in, 158–159
        after cardiac surgery, 159
        documentation of onset and termination of
            tachycardia, 158–159
    recommendations for, 158
    top priority conditions for, 157–158
    true *versus* false alarms and, 158
of ST-segment ischemia, 159–160
    nursing responsibilities in, 160–161
        differentiation of true *versus* false, 160
        lead selection for, 160
        selection of patient ST fingerprint in, 160
        setting of alarm parameters, 160
        true *versus* false alarms and, 160
    recommendations for, 159
precordial lead misplacement in, 165
precordial lead placement for, in elderly women
    with pendulous breasts, 164–165
    landmarks for, 164
quality improvement program for, 167
skills for, 166–167
skin preparation for, to reduce noisy signal and
    false alarms, 165

Electroencephalogram-based monitoring, with
    bispectral index, literature review of, 229–230

Electroencephalogram (EEG), in monitoring sedation
    level, 227–228
    physiologic basis for, 227
    relationship with bispectral index, 228

End-tidal carbon dioxide (PETCO₂), definition
    of, 217
    determinants of, 218

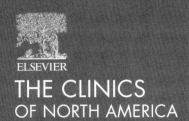

Changing Your Address?

Make sure your subscription changes too! When you notify us of your new address, you can help make our job easier by including an exact copy of your Clinics label number with your old address (see illustration below.) This number identifies you to our computer system and will speed the processing of your address change. Please be sure this label number accompanies your old address and your corrected address—you can send an old Clinics label with your number on it or just copy it exactly and send it to the address listed below.

We appreciate your help in our attempt to give you continuous coverage. Thank you.

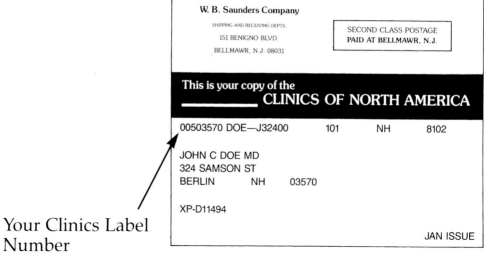

Your Clinics Label Number
Copy it exactly or send your label along with your address to:
W.B. Saunders Company, Customer Service
Orlando, FL 32887-4800
Call Toll Free 1-800-654-2452

Please allow four to six weeks for delivery of new subscriptions and for processing address changes.